Rise

The Truth Behind Epilepsy

Janine Fattaleh Diliani

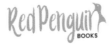

Published by Red Penguin Books

Bellerose Village, New York

Library of Congress Control Number: 2022920295

ISBN

Print 978-1-63777-334-5

Digital 978-1-63777-335-2

*To my true love Dimitri
and my guardian angel Nadine
My beloved parents Norma and Johnny
and my heroes Joseph and Johnny*

for believing in me and being my rainbow of hope

Foreword

Epilepsy is a very common chronic neurological disorder, affecting about one percent of the population worldwide. It is defined as an enduring predisposition for having epileptic seizures, which are behavioural manifestations of bursts of abnormal electrical activity in the brain. During a seizure people may or may not lose their consciousness or awareness to the environment, may have uncontrolled movements of their body, and may experience various physical or mental sensations. The exact expressions of a seizure in a certain individual depend mainly on the parts of the brain where the abnormal electrical activity originates from and on the propagation of this activity within the brain to other areas. Epilepsy has also well-recognized consequences on psychological and social aspects of the patients' lives. The main treatment of epilepsy is with medications, but about one third of the patients will continue to have seizures despite the treatment. Part of these individuals may benefit from epilepsy surgery or from electrical pacing of the abnormal brain activity.

This is a summary of what we teach medical students and young physicians about epilepsy. But Janine, in her memoir, teaches us another very important lesson about this disorder. She manages to gently take the readers to the patient's perspective of this disorder, by generously and openly letting us glimpse into the details of her life, focusing on how epilepsy has affected her over the years, either directly or through people around her. By doing this, Janine animates all the aspects of the dry medical terminology referring to epilepsy into vibrant scenes from various periods of her life. This inspiring memoir brings to life the essence of what living with epilepsy really is. As Janine's neurologist, and a physician treating people with epilepsy for many years and accompanying numerous families in their journeys alongside this disorder, through sometimes sad and sometimes happy circumstances of their lives, I read with extreme interest Janine's memoir.

Above all, this book is a heart-touching story about the maturation of a young girl in the Middle East, along with loving family members and friends, to become a brave, educated and opinionated woman, who has a significant influence on people around her. The simplicity of this story enables all readers, by identifying themselves in the character, to fully empathise with Janine, as a sometimes-rebellious adolescent, a young woman falling in love and wanting to fully experience life, and a mother devoted to carefully raising her sons. We also learn about Janine's talent for painting and poetry and about her love for sports, as well as about her deep affection for family members and friends.

The epilepsy is always there, and it seems sometimes that Janine and her loved-ones got used to it almost like getting used to a trouble-making family member, whom although you dislike, you cannot deny to. Life just goes on beside the epilepsy and despite it, somewhat in parallel to it, like living in parallel realities, which do not touch each other. One would think that after Janine stopped having seizures, she will be happy to not have anything to do with epilepsy anymore. However, the epilepsy continues to live with Janine and her family even long after she had experienced her last seizure. It is still present in their most hidden worries, but also positively emerges on the surface as beautiful thoughts and actions of Janine herself and of her relatives. Janine puts great efforts in educating various groups of the population about epilepsy and in helping other less fortunate patients cope with the disorder and reach the best treatments to alleviate it.

I think that Janine's memoir will be read with interest by people living with epilepsy, who will find themselves in the stories, coping with this unpredictable disorder, and finally in the hope for succeeding to live without it. Patients' family members and friends who care for people with epilepsy will also find interest in this book, learning from the loving response of Janine's family to her seizures and to the consequences of her disorder and medical treatment, including moody behavior at times. Finally, physicians, nurses, and other caregivers working with epilepsy patients and their families will greatly benefit from reading this book and take the opportunity to sense firsthand the obstacles this disorder poses to those who suffer from it, and on the other side – the great good that they can do in effectively treating the patients. Or at least, if effective treatment is not possible – mitigating the suffering of the patients by choosing the right medications for each patient and by advising on ways to reduce seizure frequency and severity, as well as by relating to the psychological burden of the disorder.

I am confident that scientific advances, based on research already taking place of the biological mechanisms causing epilepsy and enabling seizures' occurrence, will eventually lead to much more effective treatments of this disorder. A small artificial-intelligence-operated electrical device will likely be implanted in the brain of the patient, and it will completely prevent the development of seizures. In other cases, repair of the genetic defect leading to epilepsy will probably avoid the appearance of the disorder to start with, in susceptible individuals.

However, meanwhile, as we await these neuroscience innovations to become available for treating epilepsy patients, we can all do a lot to improve the quality of life of people who live with epilepsy and of their families. Educating the whole population on what seizures are, and on how one can help another person who has a seizure may already have a great impact on the wellbeing of people with epilepsy. This information can prevent unnecessary injuries and reduce the significant negative stigma that exists in peoples' minds about this disorder. Moreover, always seeing the person behind the epilepsy and acknowledging their qualities as human beings who are capable of contributing to society, can have a very important impact on these peoples' lives. And finally, whoever cares enough to do all that may personally benefit from meeting a friend like Janine.

~ Dana Ekstein, MD PhD, is the head of the Epilepsy Unit and chair of the Department of Neurology at Hadassah Medical Center, Jerusalem, Israel.

Chapter One

It was like something had cast a heavy shadow over my eyelids. Drifting deep into the unknown, I felt as though time didn't exist. I heard a soft monotone voice echo from a distance, though I couldn't make out what it was saying. My eyes slowly fluttered open, and dim silhouettes faded in and out of the darkness. Then, a bright light cut through the darkness, and there was a man wearing a white coat flashing a light in my eye. The voice grew louder as I began to regain consciousness. I heard a woman sniffle as if she'd been sobbing. She asked me if I knew what day it was. I was unaware of my surroundings and felt very confused. Unfamiliar faces hovered over me, looking worried. I didn't know who I was, where I was or how I'd gotten there. I felt lost in the here and now.

"This must all be a dream," I thought to myself, "a horrible nightmare." And yet, everything felt so real. I was lying on a bed, but I didn't know where. There were machines all around me, a cloth cuff was strapped around my upper arm, and an IV needle was inserted in my vein. Still disoriented, I tried to collect my thoughts, but my mind felt like a city that had just been hit by an earthquake. I slowly realized that I was in the hospital emergency room. I recognized my parents as the unfamiliar faces hovering over me earlier. Still feeling very tired and weak, I had no desire to even sit up in bed. I tried very hard to remember what had happened to bring me here, but I had no recollection at all.

I was thirteen years old and had just experienced my first grand mal seizure.

The doctors informed my parents that this disorder was incurable. Hearing this, I couldn't understand what my purpose in life was. I was terrified, imagining what it would be like to live this way forever. If my life was just going to be one of fear and misery, I may as well be in prison.

When someone commits a truly serious crime, they sometimes receive a prison sentence of twenty-five years to life. Such a harsh sentence only happens when you've done something deeply wrong, something truly unforgivable. A life sentence should never be handed down for something that wasn't your fault, something that just happened to you.

And yet, that's exactly what happened to me. I served a twenty-five-year sentence because of a medical disorder—epilepsy. I didn't ask for it. I didn't do anything to deserve it. But it was a punishment, nonetheless. It made me feel like a prisoner, with my own body as the cruelest jailer. My life became one of restrictions. I was, for a very long time, at the mercy of my disorder and had to depend on others to help me, even though what I wanted more than anything was to be independent.

My life, I'm told, was fairly normal my first few months. That changed when I was ten months old. My mom, Norma, was alone in Jerusalem with me and my sister, Nadine, while my dad, Johnny, was away on a business trip. Nadine is one year and three weeks older than me; we are like inseparable twin sisters. While my father was away, I developed a very high and very sudden fever of 41 degrees Celsius (105.8 degrees Fahrenheit). This is extremely high, particularly for a baby. My mom called my pediatrician and was instructed to immediately put me in a tub filled with room-temperature water. Then, once my temperature had dropped a little, she should bring me into the doctor's office.

My mom was supposed to join my dad, who was traveling in New York, in a few days, but after my fever, she wanted to cancel her trip. However, the pediatrician assured her that I was okay and that it would be fine for her to travel. Relieved, my mom left to meet up with my dad as planned. Nadine and I stayed with my mom's sisters, Aunt Anisa and my godmother Aunt Salwa, both of whom lived in our building.

While my parents were in New York, I had another high fever. This time, Aunt Salwa, her husband Uncle Samir, and Aunt Anisa rushed me to the hospital. I was in the hospital for three days until my fever finally went down. My parents didn't find out about this until they returned home. My aunts didn't want to worry them unnecessarily during their travels.

All these years later, I believe that whether or not my mom joined my dad on his business trip, my fever would have still happened. Epilepsy and its resulting seizures would still be my cross to bear. It didn't happen because they weren't around. Still, at the time, they blamed themselves, believing that I only had this second fever because they weren't around. It was the first—and last—time they had ever travelled together while leaving me and my sister at home.

Throughout my battle with epilepsy, my parents have been incredibly supportive. They have hearts of gold and have always been very loving, giving, and empathetic.

They've gone above and beyond for me. I owe my life to them—quite literally.

I've had seizures that last from thirty seconds to two minutes. Some have been so serious that blood flowed from my mouth, I became unconscious, my face turned blue, and my eyes rolled upward in my head. I've had bodily injuries, loss of bladder control, and bitten and bruised my lips. With my first grand mal seizure, I also had amnesia. I was, on many occasions, accused of being under the influence of alcohol or drugs. The details of each seizure or episode were somewhat different, but the underlying feeling was always the same: that of a loss of control, of being a prisoner.

Yet, through all of this, I never gave up. I constantly sought medical advice, learned more about my disorder, and tried a variety of treatments. I've seen more doctors than I care to remember, undergone hundreds of blood tests, and rode in many, many ambulances. I've had EEGs, MRIs, and CT scans and tried alternative medicine like reiki energy healing, Chinese acupuncture treatments, and attunement therapy. I've taken various types of medications, including Tegretol, Depakene, Topamax, Lamictal, and Levetirac-etam. Some succeeded in reducing the frequency of my seizures, but none completely controlled them.

After all of this, I am proud to say that I am a persistent survivor. It has taken twenty-five years—not all of them pleasant—but I have come out on the other side of my night-mare. Throughout, I've had the consistent support of my mother, father, sister, my husband Dimitri, and my children Joseph and Johnny, as well as that of extended family members and best friends. Sometimes, the kindness of strangers helped me out of the most horrific situations. There were times when people were downright cruel. Yet, I prevailed. I am here. I am married, I have children, and I have a life that I love. As a bonus, I am now a fighter in the battle to view epilepsy as a chronic disorder, not a source of stigma or shame. It's something that can be dealt with through proper medication and possibly surgery. No one should ever be ashamed of it. In fact, my first campaign slogan for epilepsy awareness was, "I have epilepsy, and I am not ashamed."

Chapter Two

I grew up female in the Middle East, an environment that is modest, traditional, and somewhat conservative when it comes to women and their expected social roles. In addition, people are often raised to think of certain illnesses and disorders as being taboo. There is so much shame associated with disorders such as epilepsy, Down's syndrome, and mental illness in our culture that some people prefer to keep their affected children at home, rather than allow them to interact with others and participate in daily life. Some may even put them in institutions where they will be cared for by others and deny these children even exist.

Epilepsy isn't a mental illness; it's a neurological disorder. Even if it were a mental illness, there shouldn't be any shame in that. However, the stigma against epilepsy is very real. A study discussed in "Factors affecting stigma of epilepsy" in *Middle East Current Psychiatry* evaluated the factors, including personality and psychological illnesses, likely to influence the social stigma associated with epilepsy in the Middle East. It found widespread attitudinal and institutional barriers and prejudices exist against people with epilepsy in education, employment, marriage, and other socioeconomic activities. Social stigma and discrimination were reported to be more devastating for people with epilepsy than the seizures themselves.

Many people in the Middle East want to hide epilepsy because they believe it is hereditary. Having a child that suffers from epilepsy might make others wonder where the child got it from. Does that mean a parent has it as well? Will any of their siblings have it, too? Will they pass it on to their children in the future? Since questions like this could come up, many parents of children with epilepsy find it easier to hide their child's condition so it won't "ruin" their siblings' chances of things like marriage.

However, epilepsy isn't always inherited or genetic. Some types of epilepsy are caused by specific events, such as a brain tumor, brain injury, severe fever, head trauma, and other causes. Anyone can develop epilepsy. It's not rare, nor is it contagious, it's not a disease. According to Epilepsy Action, if someone in the family has epilepsy, the risk of a child inheriting it depends on which type of epilepsy it is, which family member has it, and how old they were when they first developed it. The World Health Organization (WHO) estimates that around fifty million people worldwide have epilepsy, 80 percent of them in low- and middle-income countries. Epilepsy is one of the fastest-growing conditions globally, and anyone, anywhere, at any age can develop it. It is estimated that as many as 70 percent of people with epilepsy could live seizure free if diagnosed and treated properly.

During my epilepsy journey, I was told about an Arabic-language "confessions page" on Facebook in which people write about problems or issues they're going through, and others write back with words of support, comfort, and advice. The group came to my attention by a friend who told me about a young woman who wrote about her situation with epilepsy. So, I joined the group and replied to her. She initially wrote:

> *This medical disorder has haunted me since I was in middle school and prevented me from living like other girls. I am now 28 years old, and so far, no groom has come to see me [traditional marriage]. My family is against the idea that I would get married. They refused any social interactions with people. I am almost isolated from people, and no one knows me. I haven't gone to university, and I don't have friends. I see my sisters go to university, they have friends, a normal life and I'm just sitting at home simply because I am sick. Imagine missing your brother's wedding, your sister's graduation, and yearly festivities. My life is empty, I am worthless, and I am tired of living this life.*

Basically, this young woman's parents left her no hope for any kind of meaningful future. This is common in the Middle East. Many people, especially women, feel hopeless when it comes to chronic medical conditions.

I sent this young woman a message, assuring her that there is hope and that there is a surgery that could possibly help her. However, the real problem was in her parents' mentality; they didn't want to help her. I could give her all the hope in the world, but if there was no one supporting her in her daily life, it wouldn't do much good.

Still, I believe we need to break the silence surrounding such conditions and label epilepsy as what it is: a medical disorder. In Arabic, the word for epilepsy is *saraa*, which is also slang for 'crazy.' The assumption is that epilepsy is a form of mental illness. And with no one educating the community or spreading awareness about epilepsy, how could the average person know any better?

Maha is a cleaning lady who comes over once a week for a few hours. She knew I had seizures but had never witnessed one in her life. Unfortunately, her first encounter with epilepsy came about when I had a grand mal seizure while we were alone in the house together, and she was petrified. I was sitting on the couch in the living room while she was working in one of our bedrooms. She thought I was calling her and came out to see what I needed. The last thing she expected to find was me having convulsions. She couldn't understand what I was saying because she only speaks Arabic, and I was speaking English. When I came out of my seizure, I found her on the floor beside me, holding my hands and praying hysterically. She told me later that she thought I was being possessed by evil spirits, or *jinn*.

Seizures can be used as educational moments for the people around you. At one point, Maha saw me have a second grand mal seizure. My husband, Dimitri, was with me, and he called for her from the other room and asked her to go grab a towel so he could put it between my teeth. She did as he asked, but then, she just stood and watched how he handled the situation. She later told me that in that moment, instead of thinking I was possessed, her reaction was to realize how important it was to educate herself so she would know what to do if she was ever in a situation like this again. Clearly, I still felt some lingering stigma because I knew her earlier reaction was that I was possessed, but I was also glad to have helped her change her automatic reaction to seeing someone have a seizure. Now, she knew that someone having a seizure was not possessed but was in fact suffering and in the middle of a medical situation. In addition, she knew what to do in such a situation, should she ever find herself in that position again. And above all else, she could now educate others around her.

When I used to see Dr. Mark, my neurologist in Jerusalem, there were always many people sitting around me in the waiting room, and I could pick out those with epilepsy. Their heads hung low, as if they were filled with shame. My mission in life is to change that kind of thinking. Growing up with seizures, I learned everything I could about my disorder. The first time I met with Dr. Mark in Jerusalem, he was shocked by how much I knew about epilepsy. There wasn't much he could tell me except to continue monitoring my seizures and medication dosages.

Every culture has different ways of looking at various illnesses and disorders. In the Middle East, mental illness and epilepsy disorder are considered subjects that should never be discussed. As a result, many people internalize these issues out of fear of being ostracized for bringing "shame" or "dishonor" to their families and friends. Even though epilepsy is a neurological disorder, it carries the same stigma as mental illness. As a result, many people with epilepsy often hide their condition. This is harmful because it can make it harder for those struggling with epilepsy to talk openly about it and to ask for help. It's important to break the silence about mental health issues and epilepsy and talk openly about these conditions. We need to confront the stigma associated with this and label them accurately as medical disorders.

Once, a lady in the hospital said something to me about my epilepsy. She was sitting beside me in the waiting room, and we started a conversation just to kill time. We moved from one subject to another and ended up talking about epilepsy. She said to me in disbelief, "You speak so openly about your seizures!"

I answered, "Yes, I do. Am I supposed to be ashamed?" I didn't take offense at her reaction, but I also proved my point.

Almost a year ago, I had to get a dental x-ray. As soon as I entered the dentist's office, a lady in her mid-forties sitting in the waiting room greeted me. I replied with a simple hello. A minute later, she greeted me again with a lovely smile, so I once again said hello and smiled right back at her. It seemed odd, but I went along with it. While we were waiting, the power went out for about ten minutes. During that time, we ended up talking. She asked me how I was, and I told her I was fine. Then, she paused and said, "Forgive me. I like to talk a lot."

I said, "Don't worry, so do I."

I noticed that every time she spoke, her face tilted toward the ground. She was trying to explain her situation to me, but her words kept stopping and starting. She said:

I was on my way to school with my dad to take an exam, and we had a car accident. Am I bothering you, Aunt? I like to talk. Is it okay? I have metal in my head. My father is fine. We had an accident, and I was injured. I didn't take the exam.

It finally dawned on me that in her brain, she was still a child. Being the emotionally sensitive person that I am, my vision started to blur as tears filled my eyes. Something about the way she looked down at the ground every time she spoke got to me. I tried so hard to keep my tears from rolling down my face so she wouldn't notice, but they just wouldn't stop. Luckily, there was a tissue box behind the counter, so I grabbed one and kept dabbing my eyes to prevent more tears from falling. The woman continued talking about her situation and repeating things, as if she were still living in that period of her life. I realized that she might not even know what crying was because she'd shown no reactions or facial expressions to anything going on around us this whole time. The last thing I wanted was for her to think I was pitying her; I truly wasn't. I empathized with her and what she was going through. People often confuse pity and compassion because they are related emotions.

Eventually, an older man walked in and sat down across from this lady. He was looking down and scrolling through his phone. When she started talking to me again, he automatically lifted his head, squinted, and gave her a disapproving look, as if to say, "Leave her alone. You're not supposed to talk to people." From the look of it, I assumed he was her father or some other relative. I'm not a judgmental person, but the look of shame on his face upset me. He seemed ashamed to have her with him—and maybe even to have her as a child. I looked at him in disgust, as if to say, "She's talking to me, not to you." Then, I turned back to the woman and continued speaking to her.

She told me again that she had metal in her head. I tried to explain to her that I had epilepsy, that I also had metal in mine, and that I was now okay. I kept dabbing away the tears that gathered in my eyes, looking the other way so the man wouldn't see me. All I could think was, "At least give her this much. Don't make her feel like a burden to you." Thankfully, in my case, no one ever made me feel like a burden.

My name was soon called, and I went back to have my x-ray taken. The x-ray technician must have been really confused since he was looking at me straight in the face while doing the x-ray. My eyes were teary, and my nose was red.

Teaching others not to treat those with epilepsy as a burden is one of my greatest challenges and greatest desires. But I think it's working. During my first campaign, when I designed and wrote informational flyers for schools about my disorder, teachers from the schools in my neighborhood asked for more. As part of the campaign, I asked a pediatric neurologist to speak to the students, but he said I should speak instead because I can speak from personal experience. However, I can't bear the thought of standing in front of a crowd and giving a speech. Public speaking has never been my strong suit. That's why I am writing this memoir instead.

This is my story, the story of how my epilepsy started, how I've dealt with it over the years, and where I am today. I want people to know that life does go beyond epilepsy. There is hope on the other side, and it is a life that is definitely worth living. Hopefully, my story will provide hope to others who suffer from this disorder or those supporting loved ones with epilepsy.

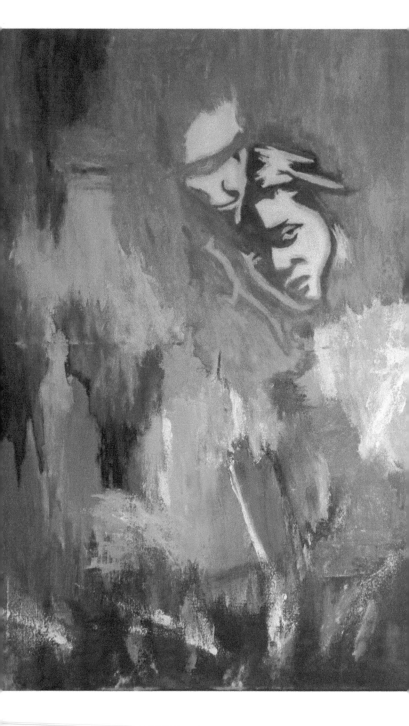

Step Outside

She smiles to the world and shares her warmth
with jewel-like eyes that sparkle when she speaks

She follows her heart blindly and loves with compassion
with pure innocent eyes that dazzle when she speaks

She hears imminent storm tides and feels one's sadness
with true heartfelt eyes that listen when she speaks

She embraces sore wounds and shields invisible scars
with honest mystic eyes that comfort when she speaks

She stepped outside herself whilst chaos stirred her soul
with dry teary eyes that sparkle when she speaks

Epilepsy affected everyone in my family, not just me. I'm fortunate to have such wonderful family and friends, as they ended up being one of the most important parts of my journey over the next twenty-five years.

I had a typical childhood and teenage existence. I was the ultimate tomboy, played all the sports I could, and hung out with my girlfriends at every opportunity. However, all that changed when I had my first memorable seizure at the age of thirteen in Jeddah, Saudi Arabia. I was going to a volleyball tournament with my team, and as I stepped off the school bus, I had my first grand mal seizure.

This is how my classmate and friend Jeanne described that seizure:

> I remember the bus being cold with the air conditioner on. The girls were all excited and nervous about the volleyball competition. Then Janine got out ahead of me and within a few steps, she fell to the ground and started convulsing. The girls all screamed and ran, and I went into what I now call paramedic mode, (as I have used my first aid training a number of times to help others. If I could change how we teach children, it would be to include first aid and mental health first aid).
>
> I remember she wasn't conscious of what was going on, and I grabbed a backpack to put under her head and pulled her tongue from her throat--I got into trouble for that by the school and my dad, because they said she could have bitten my finger off.
>
> I yelled at someone to go and get the coach, can't remember his name, and he came running and then it was a blur. I do remember her being in the school first aid room with the nurse.
>
> We were forced to play volleyball, but most of us were

too concerned about her to care about the game! I think
we lost, too.

All I remember from that day is waking up in the ER confused and unable to recognize my parents. They kept asking me questions, trying to remind me of who I was, who they were, and where I was. I was clueless until, like a light-bulb turning on in my brain, I suddenly remembered who I was and who they were and answered them. What a relief that was for them! However, I was still confused, as I wasn't aware of all that had happened until later that evening when they finally told me.

After my seizure on the school bus, the school secretary called my mom and told her that I had been taken to the hospital because I had a seizure on the way to the volleyball game. My mom, startled, called my dad, and they both rushed to the hospital to see me and to find out exactly what had happened. This is what my mom recalls from that day:

I had the shock of my life. All kinds of thoughts were racing inside my head. How could this be, she was fine this morning, what went wrong, why did this happen to her. I panicked and called Johnny and told him this horrible news. I was so afraid; I couldn't believe this was happening. I grabbed my purse and rushed down to meet him at the entrance of the hotel. The ride to the hospital felt like forever. I couldn't wait to see her.

There she was lying on the bed, and I rushed over to hug her, but she didn't recognize me. Johnny and I were terrified and asked to see the doctor. The neurologist sat us down and explained the situation. He said that she had suffered from a Tonic-Clonic (Grand Mal) seizure, but she was okay. Okay, I said? She doesn't know who we are, how can she be, okay? He told us that seizures can affect

occurred that day, and the medication dosage I was taking at the time. It was important to note medication dosage, because that helped me track whether my current dosage was sufficient for the number of seizures I was having each month or whether it was time for my neurologist to increase the dosage or maybe even change my medication completely.

From these logs, I learned that my triggers included fear of death, nervousness, anger, feeling cold or upset, and my monthly period, due to the fluctuation of hormones. However, this doesn't mean that they didn't occur at other times. Sometimes, my seizures came out of the blue. But at least I could try to prevent them from happening as much as I could.

In addition to keeping a close eye on me, my family also made sure I didn't get cold, upset, or angry, and they all knew to never share any bad news with me, especially when it had to do with death. I occasionally heard them hushing each other or caught them winking or making silent communications with their eyes, as if they were about to accidentally mention something they shouldn't in front of me. They were always on high alert worrying that these things could cause me to have a seizure. As frustrating as that was for me, I knew their intentions were good.

Having one seizure doesn't mean you have epilepsy; having two or more seizures does. Also, there are many different types of seizures. I suffered from two different types of seizures.

The first type is called complex partial seizures. This is when a seizure begins in one area or side of the brain, most commonly in the temporal lobe or frontal lobe. When I had this kind of seizure, I would appear to be unresponsive and unaware of my surroundings and had involuntary actions, such as lip smacking, rubbing my hands, and, at times, wandering. These seizures were often mistaken for a psychiatric disorder or drug or alcohol abuse. They were sometimes preceded by an aura, which served as a warning, and then lasted for anywhere from thirty seconds to one or two minutes.

The other type of seizure I had was a tonic-clonic seizure, also known as a grand mal seizure. This type of seizure affects large areas of the brain. With these seizures, I would lose consciousness and experience severe muscle contraction. My body would tense up, my fists would close, and convulsions would shake my entire body, causing violent jerking of all my muscles. For me, these seizures lasted less than two minutes, and upon regaining consciousness, I would be confused, disoriented, and without any memory of what had transpired. Luckily, my seizures never exceeded two minutes and did not require medical help. Only if a seizure lasts longer than five minutes is it necessary to call an ambulance for medical help. After these seizures, I felt tired and weak. They were extremely draining.

My parents and Nadine quickly learned to recognize when a seizure was about to occur. The best warning sign was that I would start to rub my hands together and smack my lips. However, at first, there were no consistent warning signs. Any unusual sensation or feeling, experience, or movement that just seems odd or different is known as an 'aura.' It's a warning that occurs before a seizure. However, there isn't always an aura before a seizure. Sometimes, my seizures just happened.

Personally, I felt like the aura itself was a horrible experience. Those automatic movements were always accompanied by an awful, indescribable feeling that is difficult to put into words. It often started with a strange feeling of impending doom in the pit of my stomach and a queasy, tingling, unpleasant sensation. In those moments, I was absolutely terrified and felt an urgent need to get to safety. Everything became strange to me in an awful frightening way. That feeling continued and rushed across my chest, up through my esophagus, and then out over my tongue, carrying with it the strangest taste. That's when the seizure occurred. I've been told that, occasionally, during a grand mal seizure, I seemed to have shortness of breath and chest pains. I would unconsciously clutch my hand to my chest and mutter in distress that my chest hurt. Of course, I can't recall any of that.

After the first few years, my auras continued before a seizure, but the lip smacking and hand rubbing stopped, so there was no longer a consistent warning sign for my family. Instead, they had to look for a sudden change in me, such as my speech becoming heavier or going blank in the face or losing track of what I was saying and starting to slow down or mumble. These were the only external signs, and the horrible, frightening feelings inside me made it almost impossible for me to speak out and warn others around me.

On occasion, I experienced unusual auras. For example, one time, I was sitting with a friend, having a conversation, when suddenly, I saw her face slowly split into square cubes and everything became strange, still, and very unfamiliar. It was like there was a distortion of time and my visual perception was off. This was accompanied by the horrible, frightening feeling that always accompanied an aura. At other times, when my aura started, the person I was with no longer seemed familiar to me. I could no longer relate to anything around me; it all became strange. The feeling of being totally disconnected from the world around me was like an unpleasant out-of-body sensation. It was painful and frightening.

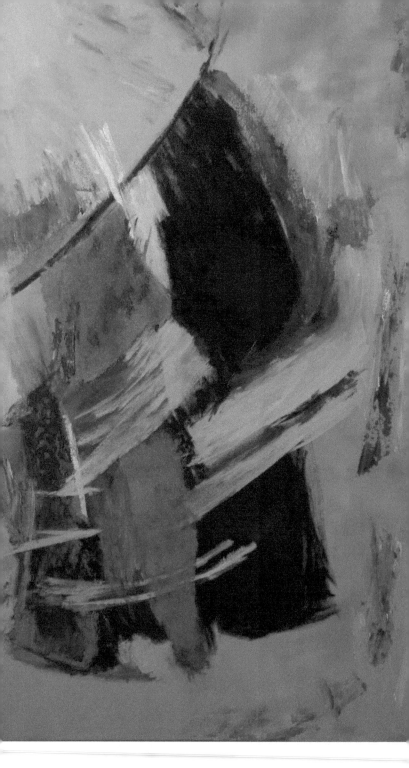

Chaos

I can feel it heading this way
a destructive opposing force
I can feel it heading this way
a twister taking its course

I can hear rapid motion sounds
of confusion, panic, and fear
I can hear swift current waves
raging to make ends meet

I can feel its presence... Chaos

During my seizures, I always repeated the same words out loud "Say something nice, or say I love you"—over and over again. A few years into my epilepsy journey, I also began asking for a hug or a kiss and calling for Nadine or saying, "I love you, Nadine," regardless of who was helping me. This remained a constant throughout the rest of my journey. When people who had never seen a seizure before heard me say this, they were often confused or thought I was crazy. And really, who wouldn't think I was crazy? Even though it is so wrong to call someone crazy, or saraa in Arabic slang. People can say what they are going to say or think what they are going to think. But what I'd like is to see its medical term labeled differently. Label epilepsy as what it is, a disorder. Not being crazy. People are already unaware, and it's no wonder why they think the way they do when epilepsy is labeled crazy. People will naturally believe or misunderstand that if you have epilepsy, you are crazy.

After all, seizures don't always look or sound like they do in movies or on TV. Eventually though, they'd realize, "Oh, she really does need me to say something nice because something strange is happening to her."

Try to envision yourself saying this to a complete stranger, which did happen occasionally when my friends and family weren't around. I've had many seizures in public and had strangers help me. Those were the seizures I worried about the most, because anything is possible during an aura and seizure. Since you're not aware of what's going on during a seizure, you're at the mercy of those around you and you can't protect yourself from people with bad intentions. Just thinking about such situations scared me, and that fear always lurked in the background of my mind. If I was waiting my turn at the bank, my thoughts would start to drift toward what might happen if I were to have a seizure now. Would I fall to the ground and become unconscious? Would the people around me freak out? Would someone know how to help me if I started to have convulsions? Or, if I was at an ATM, would someone steal my purse or try to hurt me in some way? Sometimes, while going down an escalator, I'd worry about having a seizure and falling down the moving stairs. These kinds of thoughts could easily spiral out of control and get pretty ugly.

Chapter Four

There's a common saying I've seen online: "A woman without her sister is like a bird without wings."

My sister Nadine was my biggest support when we were young. Being so close in age, we were always together in school, during outings, and with friends. She was always there for me, she took care of me when needed, and she never turned her back on me or complained about me. I looked up to her, and even today, she is still one of my greatest supports, my backbone. She never made me feel like a burden. She was also always very honest with me and never beat around the bush. She wouldn't lie to me to make me feel better. I'd vent to her, and she helped me carry the weight of my situation. She never pushed me away; instead, she always gave me the best advice. In doing so, she gave me self-confidence. She helped me gain strength and believe in myself, rather than feel like there was something wrong with me or that I needed special treatment. She sacrificed a lot for me, and that is the purest and most selfless way to love someone. I think that's why I always called out to her during my seizures—because she was always there for me. She gave me the greatest gift while growing up: an ever-

panic attack is. I didn't back then, but that's how they seemed. She did panic, then she needed comfort and she was scared. During her seizure, she always needed to hold someone's hand until it passed and know that they cared. They were always the same. I hadn't seen another grand mal seizure like that until we lived in Miami, and she had another in her townhouse kitchen. She, Nadine, and I were in the kitchen talking and she dropped next to the fridge. Nadine knew what to do and when she came around, she was ok. By then, she was on medication and her sister knew exactly what to do. I remember the constant worry on her mom's face, the regular medication on the bedside table, but she was never afraid, and she never stopped doing what she enjoyed. I think, looking back, I finally know why she always had Simon, their driver, with her, waiting for her, always there. Just in case. If that was the reason, it was a smart move by her mom and dad.

When I was diagnosed with epilepsy, my parents informed my school, the Continental British International School in Jeddah, where I spent my middle school and high school years, of my medical condition. The school administration and teachers were all very supportive and never treated me differently from the other students. I was not given any special education or treatment, and I never felt like I needed it. During my time there, I was elected student *counselor* and continued to play sports, to the extent that I needed two knee arthroscopic surgeries—a surgical procedure that treats damaged cartilage in the knee to lessen friction in the joint—in my late teens. I graduated from The Continental School in 1994 at the age of sixteen.

Mrs. Awan was my favorite teacher, and she was also a great support for me when my life first turned upside down.

We stayed in touch after I graduated, and she agreed to share her recollection of watching me grow up in middle school and in high school:

I was Janine's teacher at Continental School, in math, although that wasn't her favorite subject. I met her in 1990, when she was thirteen. She was always determined to succeed. What I remember most is her athleticism and sense of fairness. I chose her to be head of West House, one of the four sports teams we had at school. She was one of the most reliable, responsible, and physically gifted students I had.

One day after a netball game, I saw her on the concrete floor, shaking quite a bit with spit coming out of her mouth and unaware of her surroundings. As a group of concerned schoolmates gathered, I realized she was having a seizure. I turned her head to one side, and we gently held her arms down. It was over quickly. When it was over, she was surprised to find herself on the floor with many curious eyes looking at her. She had no recollection of the event. But in her usual strong way, she brushed it off and went on as usual. I felt it was my duty to tell her family. Initially they didn't take it well.

What I want to say is that Janine must have felt it before that, but she never let it contain her as a person. Once she knew what it was, she was even more determined to carry on as normal even to surpass her past achievements. She was never embarrassed, scared, or shy. That I thought was a brilliant quality. She was determined to conquer it. She embraced it, learned to control it, and to live a better life in spite of it. She was elected student counselor in her senior year.

She is an inspiration to all with any shortcoming. I

met her recently in Dubai and it was a great pleasure to see her. I wanted to cry. I was so happy.

I often felt like I was a burden on family and friends, though I know that's not how they felt, and they never made me feel that way. And yet, I constantly worried, "What if I have a seizure now? What if it's a bad one that'll be embarrassing for me and for them? Why should they have to deal with all this, even if they say they're okay with it? They shouldn't have to constantly think about all the what-ifs themselves. Maybe they don't want to be seen with me. Maybe I'll ruin their outing. Who would want to take on the responsibility of having me along? I'm just a liability." These thoughts were always present in my mind, no matter where I was or who I was with.

Aside from my fear of being embarrassed and wondering what people were saying or thinking about me, I had to deal with the fact that most people do not know how to help someone who's having a seizure, especially if caught off-guard. There are many things about seizures that people just aren't aware of. For instance, whenever I had a grand mal seizure, my tongue would flip backward toward my tonsils, and most people's first, automatic fear was that I'd swallow my tongue. They'd panic and focus on controlling the tongue, often by putting something in my mouth, which is actually quite dangerous. However, there is no such thing as swallowing your tongue; it's impossible. There is a small piece of tissue in the human mouth, which sits behind the teeth and below the tongue and keeps the tongue in place, even during a seizure. Most people don't know that, though. The only real concern was that my tongue might block my airway and suffocate me. To prevent this, people who knew me had me lie down and turn onto my side so that when my tongue flipped backward during the attack, I could still breathe. The person having a seizure is indeed helpless, but the person helping them is just as helpless if it's their first time seeing a seizure.

That said, the idea of being helpless has always been foreign to my family. They never really understood the meaning of the word. They did everything in their power to help me, no matter the circumstances.

Not every disability is visible; epilepsy is one of those. Just because someone with epilepsy looks just fine, it doesn't mean they are. There were many occasions when I was going about my day, living my life, when I suddenly had a seizure. In addition, the medications that I took to control my seizures severely affected my behavior toward others, often causing them to misjudge me.

One time, I was invited to a pre-wedding lunch at my cousin Hiba's fiancé's house in Amman, Jordan, with my parents and Nadine. In addition to my extended family, there were lots of other people there. I was getting my food, trying to blend in with everyone else, when I suddenly felt an aura coming on. Within seconds, my plate fell to the tiled floor and shattered into a million pieces. The food was all over my clothes and on the floor. I was so embarrassed, not just for me but also for Hiba. I wished the ground would just swallow me up. My parents, Nadine, and my dad's sisters, Aunt Alice, Aunt Nina, and Aunt Janet, took me aside and hovered over me, reassuring me that everything was okay, that nothing bad had happened, and that it was no big deal. Oh, but it was to me! Here I was, trying to make a good impression, and this happened! So many thoughts were racing through my mind, especially about Hiba and how she must've felt about all this commotion. It's really hard when you feel like every eye in the room is on you. You can't help but wonder what people are thinking. It was also the first time Hiba, my aunts, and my Uncle Tony had ever witnessed a grand mal seizure.

As if one humiliation wasn't enough, the same thing happened during another large gathering at my Aunt Anisa's house in Jerusalem.

Despite these challenges, my family always made an effort to include me in special events and daily activities. My parents wanted me to live as normal a life as possible. My father recalls:

I have two Jewels, Nadine and Janine. We weren't familiar with epilepsy as we don't have it in the family. The first thing we did when we found out about Janine's epilepsy was to comfort her and take her to the best neurologist in Jeddah SA where I was based at the time.

As Janine got older, she had to remember to take her medication on time. Norma and I still today ask her if she's taken it, but she relies on herself. She was confident not to be obsessed with her disorder. She lived her life normally at school and at home. We always encouraged her to lead her life as normal. It is a father's worst nightmare to watch his child suffer from any medical illness. It was very painful for me to see her have a seizure while I couldn't do anything about it. We never lost hope and always tried to find solutions and treatments. Unfortunately, nothing worked. That didn't stop us, we continued trying and never gave up. My advice to parents of kids with epilepsy is to be patient, never lose hope, love them unconditionally and work with a neurologist and get the right advice.

When Dimitri asked for her hand in marriage, it was moral to tell him how severe her seizures were, even though he already knew about Janine's medical disorder.

We eventually came to find out that the only option that could work was the brain surgery in the right frontal lobe of her brain. This would give Janine an 85% chance to be seizure free. After many discussions we opted for the surgery, which she did on 10/29/2015. Since then, she has been seizure free, but she still has to take medicine daily. That was one of the best days of my life with many tears of joy. I thank God almighty and St. Charbel, for listening to our daily prayers and protecting her during the surgery and always.

Chapter Five

Being a teenager is already difficult, so epilepsy was the last thing I needed to add to that experience. Even if it is well-controlled, epilepsy can be a huge problem. When I was first diagnosed, I was afraid of being isolated or bullied. I wondered, "What will the other students say about me? Will I scare them away? Will they laugh about it later and make fun of my actions during the seizure?" I was also worried that I wouldn't be able to do the things I wanted to do, like play sports and have a normal social life with my friends. I constantly lived in fear and doubt, never knowing when the next seizure might strike. That alone was a nightmare. The fact that there was nothing I could do to stop the seizure when I felt it coming felt like the ultimate defeat.

At first, I thought that epilepsy would make me stand out and that people would treat me differently because of it. I was constantly anxious. But with time, I realized that these were all misconceptions that existed only in my head. Most students at school probably didn't even know I had epilepsy, no one was watching me like a hawk, and I wasn't in the spotlight all the time. That realization gave me the courage to live a normal life and the strength to accept that this was a disorder I just had to live with.

It really helps if you try to take epilepsy in stride and not feel like it's too big a deal. Then, it's much more likely that your friends will regard it the same way. That's what happened with me. Sure, my friends were terrified at first, but they eventually learned how to help me and what to do during a seizure. They got over their fear, and we felt comfortable hanging out together. My seizures were never a subject of discussion among my friends; they were irrelevant.

Lara has been one of my best friends since my early teens. We met in Jerusalem, but we never lived in the same country. Our friendship grew stronger through letters, long distance phone calls, and short visits. Decades later, when I moved to Jerusalem, knowing she lived there was my greatest comfort and blessing. She recalls:

> *The first time I saw Janine have a seizure, I stood frozen in fear while Nadine was helping her get through it. I remember she told me what I had to do if it ever happened, but it wasn't what I imagined. It was a scary experience, I had never seen someone have a seizure before hers, it's not something you see everyday. But then, I knew what to expect and exactly what to do. I remember our long-distance phone calls, constant letters in the mail and such good times we've spent together. She never circled her life around her seizures, and even though she was a strong person I would always worry about her and wanted to make sure she stayed safe.*

Another one of my best friends to this day is Nisreen. We also met in our teens, though we never lived in the same country or attended the same school. Our relationship grew stronger through phone calls, letters, and pit stops in Jordan while crossing over to Jerusalem twice a year. Of all my friends, Nisreen saw all my phases and sides during my journey because our paths crossed the most. But she always stood by my side. Here are some of Nisreen's recollections:

One of my memories is when we were out with some girls, and I recall being protective of Janine. I remember what used to happen when she was having a seizure. We'd be sitting and she'd start to talk quite fast. She would need consolation; I would have to hold her hand and hug her and keep telling her I love you. I felt compassion. It never bothered me or upset me. I wanted to help her, to make it all go away. I wanted to shield her from the world. I knew people wouldn't understand. I didn't want them to judge her.

I felt from the beginning, and I still feel today, that fate had it that we would meet. I was very lucky to have met her. Had I not met her I would never have seen the world she had to navigate, and it changed me so much. I've gained such growth and compassion. Seeing first-hand, epilepsy and seizures and how they happen and how they made her and how she handled it affected me positively. I have more empathy, and I've grown as a human. I'm very thankful for it now, I do feel so different from many people I know because of her, the strength she always showed that inspired me.

I'm so very lucky and blessed to have had all these amazing, supportive best friends in my life. I can't imagine what my life as a teenager and young adult suffering from seizures would have been like without them. My friends' support and belief in me gave me the power to choose: was I going to live a full, normal life, or was I going to hide behind

worked almost 95 percent of the time because music distracts me and calms my mind. While listening to music, I'm not as focused on the motion around me. Even today, unless I'm the one driving, you'll always find me wearing an earphone in one ear, just to take my mind off the road.

Men, usually adolescents or young adults, often harassed women in cars who had drivers. They would tail these cars, pull up beside them, and flash their mobile numbers or try to talk to the women. For this reason, most cars had fabric curtains over the backseat windows to prevent other men from seeing inside the car.

Being teenagers, we were frequently harassed this way. Once, Nada and I were heading to her house after school. While waiting at a traffic light, a guy came up to our car, opened the back door, and tossed in a piece of paper with his mobile number on it, scaring us half to death. Then, he started tailing us. I told Nada's driver to take us to my house instead because the guy following us wouldn't think that my house was in a hotel, and he'd drive away.

Restaurants had a 'family section' and a 'men's section.' If family groups or groups of women wanted to dine together, they sat in the family section. Men could only enter the family section if they were with an immediate family member of the opposite sex, such as a sister, wife, or daughter.

Shops and restaurants were required to close during the Muslim prayer times. If you were inside an establishment before prayer time, you could either leave before prayer began or you'd have to stay inside until after prayer time ended; you were not allowed to leave before then. We were occasionally caught in that situation and had to decide whether to stay or go, depending on what was more convenient.

I once had a frightful experience with a *mutawa* during

such a closure. A few of the girls on our school basketball team decided to get a burger at Wendy's one evening. There were six of us, and we all arrived at Wendy's at about the same time, each with our own driver, plus a housemaid who, like Simon for me, was always with one of the girls as an escort for safety reasons. We planned to eat dinner during the time the restaurant was closed for evening prayer.

This Wendy's was located on a very busy street, so there was always commotion and several *mutawas* around, but during prayer time, it wasn't as busy. Usually, restaurants and shops were almost empty during this time, so it was the perfect opportunity to feel comfortable in our own quiet space. We were all wearing abayas and cheerfully entered the family section together, though we were careful not to be too loud, so we wouldn't attract attention. The entrance to the men's section was right beside the entrance to the family section, which made it easy for men to harass women. We placed our orders, and then went to sit upstairs. Soon, we were eating and having a good time; the restaurant was practically ours.

Suddenly, we heard stomping footsteps coming up the stairs. The next thing we knew, there was a *mutawa* and a uniformed policeman heading straight toward us. We all panicked. Since I took every opportunity I could to not wear an abaya, mine was thrown somewhere behind me on the bench we were sitting on. There was only one other couple sitting at the other end of the restaurant, so I felt comfortable taking it off. The girls quickly squeezed close to me and started covering my legs with my abaya, since I was in shorts and didn't have enough time to put it on. We were scared, yet unable to stop giggling because my abaya wouldn't stay still on my lap; it just kept sliding down.

The *mutawa* and policeman weren't amused and started scolding us, but we pretended that we couldn't

married, I put my medication in my wedding ring. If I was ever in doubt about whether I'd taken my medication, all I had to do was look at my fingers and check my rings.

Of course, I can't say I never missed a dose. After all, it's only human to occasionally forget a dose or take it late. There were a few times when I dozed off and forgot to take off my rings. When I realized my mistake, I'd take the missed dose immediately and then delay the following dose by four hours, as my doctor instructed. But for the most part, my 'rings system' worked well because my rings were important to me. Find something that's important to you, and you'll almost never forget your medicine.

My parents encouraged me to do as many things as possible while also recognizing and managing the risks. They allowed me to stay out at night, go on a ski trip with my school to Santa Fe in Switzerland. Lina also went on that trip, and we had a blast. Even now, when I look at the photos we took together, it brings back such fond memories. I also traveled with my friends to Spain and sometimes to Lebanon during our spring or summer vacations. This helped me make a successful transition into adulthood because I learned that epilepsy was *my* disorder, not theirs. I started to create my own lifestyle, make the right choices, take responsibility for my actions, and learn how to take care of myself. I wouldn't be where I am today if it weren't for my parents' and Nadine's support while growing up.

Epilepsy can also aggravate or create behavioral problems. I used to have mood swings, outbursts, and other behavioral issues, but they accepted it, embraced me with their unconditional love, and always advocated for me. They knew that I was experiencing side effects from my medication, so they tolerated it. Epilepsy was a part of me, but I never let it define me.

I always tried to look on the bright side of things, but I

couldn't escape my negative perspective on things related to my seizures, especially my thoughts on life. My medications only made this worse. Yes, I smiled, laughed, enjoyed life as much as possible, and did the things I wanted to do, but there was still so much sadness and pain hidden beneath the surface. No one could see that, though; all they could see was the anger, outbursts, and negativity. Some may have judged me for it, but my loved ones tolerated it. People don't change at their core, even when veiled in darkness. I always have and still do give people the benefit of the doubt because I'm not a judgmental person. I don't try to find people's faults because everyone is fighting their own battles. Living with epilepsy taught me that there's a lot more to people than what meets the eye.

After my surgery, I had a more positive outlook on life. I learned how to turn a negative into a positive and how much brighter life could be once I allowed it to be. It was impossible to feel this way while I was fighting my battle with epilepsy; my medications only made the situation worse. During my fight, I never even thought of trying to see the world in a more positive light. For that matter, I didn't really want to. All I could focus on was what my seizures were doing to me.

I made the best of my situation, but perhaps putting effort into turning the negatives into positives might've helped. It wouldn't have made my seizures go away, but it would've shed some light on my darkness. I counted my blessings every single day, which is a very positive thing to do, and I appreciated everything I had in life. But that still wasn't enough to make me a positive person. I was still a very negative person, and that tends to push people away. People with negative energy attract negative people, so you're basically two peas in a pod. Over the years, I've found that when I'm around people who are full of positive

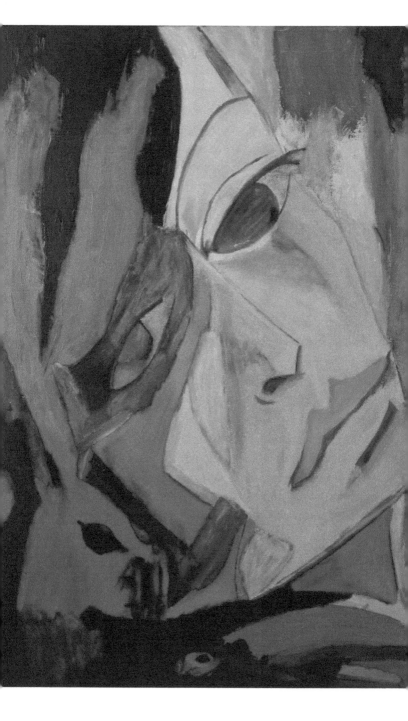

Beauty and the Beast

Gripped onto steel bars with nothing to set me free
empowers demons that are blinding my colorful soul
Sheltering them paralyzes my heart that hungers to heal
where it'll be too late to find what I'm searching for

Loud screams are trapped inside my head
which deny me from guiding my inner strength
Locking myself behind an iron cell
has carved a hole that yearns to weld

Thunder roars at me until my angry soul awakes
entices violence that my inner self awaits
Releasing my screams out into open air
where deviant behavior becomes my daring glare

Curl into a shielded soul
that'll float above a burning flame
Depriving me of closure that I've longed for
but shelters my wounds that reside deep in my soul

Chapter Eight

I was determined not to let epilepsy run my life. I wasn't going to let it control me. If anything, I was going to control it. This meant leading an ordinary life and doing things without letting my unfortunate disorder limit me. Even if they were frightening or something I didn't exactly look forward to, I forced myself to charge forward.

Lina, Kerry, and I all ended up studying together at the University of Miami. Being so far away from our families, we lived in the same residential compound and took very good care of each other. One of the craziest things I ever did was with them.

They decided to go on an ejection seat ride at a fair. This is essentially a reverse-bungee jump that is akin to a slingshot. It has two steel towers with a bungee cord connected to each steel tower. Two passengers are secured inside a cage, which is released into the air from the loading base. It reaches a maximum speed of 97 kilometers per hour (60 miles per hour) and a maximum height of 45 meters (148 feet). The caged cell shoots from its loading base, spins in the air a few times as it launches skyward, and then comes shooting down again, giving the passengers an adren-

eye on me, and I was still having an average of four or five seizures a week.

I started seeing Dr. Thomas every month. He had me do a blood test at every visit and changed the dosage of my medication based on the results. Tegretol can damage the liver, which is why I required a monthly blood test. He wanted to keep my Tegretol dosage at the therapeutic level, where it was high enough to have the intended effect, but low enough so as not to damage my liver. If my blood test showed that liver damage was occurring, he'd decrease my dosage; if there wasn't any liver damage, he'd increase it. That's all he ever did. He never even looked at my seizure log. And I was still having four or five seizures a week. I didn't even realize that the medicine wasn't preventing seizures. I didn't consider that there might be medicines out there that could actually control my seizures or possibly even prevent them from happening at all. Why would I think? I wasn't a doctor. What did I know? The Internet barely existed at the time, and my first impulse wasn't to go out and research things at the library. Now, doing some basic research online is almost everyone's automatic first step. It helps to have everything you need to know right at your fingertips.

It wasn't until my Aunt Anisa told my parents that she knew a lady with a different type of epilepsy who was taking Tegretol, and it prevented her from having seizures entirely that I realized Dr. Thomas wasn't doing his job properly. He seemed more interested in giving me pills and getting me out the door than actually exploring my problem and finding a solution that would truly help. I decided to find another neurologist, Dr. Patrick.

At our first meeting, I stormed into his office. I was already angry before the appointment even started. I immediately announced, "If you're going to give me Tegretol, just tell me now, and I'll leave."

Luckily, he was used to this type of behavior. Outbursts of anger is a common side effect of anti-epileptic medications. He told me to sit down and spent a good hour talking with me. As we talked, he took notes on the long white sheet of paper that covered the examining table. He made multiple line charts on the paper and used them to explain all the different anti-epileptic medications available, breaking them down by their side effects and which ones he thought might be best for me to try.

He reduced my Tegretol dosage and added a different type of anti-epileptic medication, Depakene. I had to be weaned off the Tegretol gradually. You can't just stop taking them overnight. A few months later, when I was able to get off the Tegretol entirely, he added another type of anti-epileptic medication, Topamax. He said the combination of Depakene and Topamax would control my seizures better— or maybe even fully. Dr. Patrick warned me that Depakene might cause hair loss, and he recommended that I start taking vitamins to help prevent that. So, I started taking hair, skin, and nails vitamins, and I've continued taking them ever since. Generally, people shed between fifty and one hundred single hairs per day; shedding hair isn't the same as hair loss. Hair loss is when you have handfuls of hair falling out at a time and bald spots. Luckily, this never happened with me, and my hair remained very healthy.

Dr. Patrick also had me undergo a twenty-four-hour electroencephalograph (EEG) monitoring test to identify when and where a seizure was happening and to record the brain's electrical activity surrounding the episode. They attached electrodes to my scalp with enough glue to ensure that they'd remain in place, especially when I slept. When I felt a seizure coming on, I was supposed to press a button on the machine wrapped around my waist, which connected to the electrodes with wires. As fate would have it, I had a seizure that night while I was asleep and pressed the button too late for it to record the full seizure.

He also did an MRI and a regular EEG, which showed that my seizures were 99.9 percent located in the right front temporal lobe. This meant that it was safe to operate, should we go that route. However, the surgery to address my type of seizure was still brand-new, so I'd essentially be a guinea pig. At the time, only two or three patients had undergone this type of surgery. He preferred to continue trying to control my seizures with medication and leave surgery as an option for the future.

Once I was on the two new medicines, I could feel the difference almost immediately. It was like a weight had been taken off my shoulders. Some of my fear and anxiety melted away. The constant feeling of cloudiness hovering over me vanished. These two medications helped reduce my seizures down to just three or four a month. I just wish it hadn't taken six years.

Chapter Nine

All these medications had different side effects, as most medicines do. Many of these side effects were similar and included mood swings, depression, blurred vision, double vision, nausea, outbursts of anger, self-harm, suicidal thoughts, tremors, crying, and acne, just to name a few. Topamax, my newest medication, had additional side effects of weight loss and feelings of paranoia. As horrible as those two additional side effects were, switching to Topamax and Depakene helped reduce the frequency of my seizures for the first time. It gave me a renewed sense of hope.

My weight dropped drastically to forty-two kilograms (ninety-two pounds) and stayed that low the whole time I was on Topamax. Regardless of what I ate, my weight remained the same. The smallest jeans I could find were still too big for me, and my ribs and spine stuck out. For some people taking Topamax, this is an advantage. It's an easy way to lose weight. In fact, I once saw on *Good Morning America tv show* that Topamax was being sold on the black market as a weight loss drug. I didn't think it was worth it, though; my mental health suffered too much.

I had frequent thoughts of suicide, a very common side effect of anti-epileptic drugs. I was constantly assailed by these dark thoughts. It was almost impossible to silence them. They distorted my perceptions, clouded my thinking, and led me to impulsive behavior. It was frightening. What's worse, these thoughts would appear during my most vulnerable moments or when I was very miserable. When this happened, I would sink in a whirlpool of dark thoughts that was difficult to escape from. I felt trapped by my own thoughts. Being trapped in your mind is an awful feeling. I was constantly feeding my pain, telling myself things like, "I'm worthless. I can't live like this anymore. I hate my life. Nothing's working. I just want to die." Rather than challenging my dark thoughts, I allowed myself to drown in them. And the more I fed my pain, the more difficult it was to escape. I kept digging and digging, and the deeper I got, the harder it was to crawl back out. I was trapped in a bottomless pit, a prison of my own making.

Regardless of how miserable I was, I knew that I could never take my own life. I would only be harming those who loved me, and I couldn't be that selfish—another trait my parents taught me. My love and faith helped me fight to live and quiet those compelling suicidal thoughts. My family and best friends were such a great support to me that I didn't want to let them down. I didn't want to be remembered as a quitter because that's not who I am. I'd worked too hard and built myself up too well. I wasn't going to give that all up. I chose to be a fighter, and I was determined not to lose. But at times, it was hard.

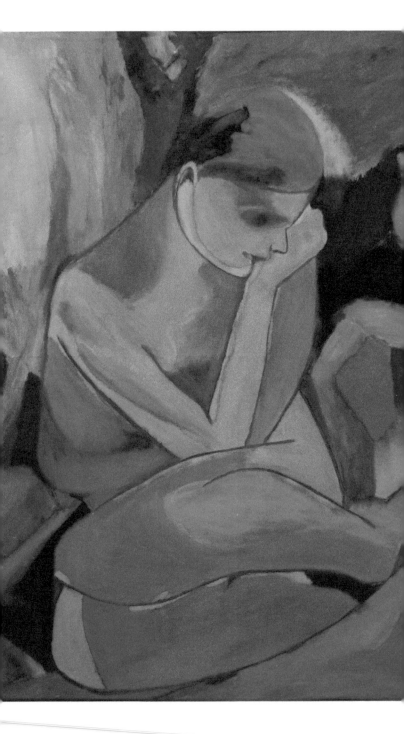

Break Free

Fight your demons and put them to sleep,
where they can no longer poison your soul
Inviting them to stay will make them your shadow
and you can never outrun what you stow

Swallow your emotions and keep fighting,
giving yourself enough space to breathe
Where strength has become your trophy,
and you know you've survived the ordeal

Anger goes away when you lock the door,
where love has proven to conquer all
Trying to change what can't be undone,
you'll struggle in the days that are yet to come

During my time in university, I was determined not to let epilepsy get the better of me, so I went out and had fun doing all the things that typical university students do.

One time, at a nightclub, I asked a waiter for water so I could take my evening dose of medication. I had forgotten to take it at home earlier that evening, but I always had some in my purse in case of an emergency. Missing a dose of my medication could provoke a seizure, and I wanted to avoid that, especially in a club.

There was a man sitting next to me, and he saw me take my medication. He apparently thought I was just popping some kind of pill for fun because he said, "You know, I can have you arrested for something like this." Then, he flashed his badge at me. Apparently, he was an off-duty cop. Luckily, he was one of the good guys. There are people who would have taken advantage of me in that situation, but he didn't. I showed him my medic alert bracelet and explained that I was taking my medication, and that was that. Still, I learned an important lesson that day: never take my medication in a nightclub.

Over the years, I've known pain, fear, confusion, frustration, depression, tears, and the loss of self. But I've always been a warrior. I fought to keep my life moving forward. Of course, you should take my advice with a grain of salt, since I don't know you and your circumstances, but remember that life will always throw curveballs at you. Never let your life stagnate. Force yourself out of monotony, challenge your limits, and most importantly, be unpredictable. Above all else, always remember who or what in your life makes you want to keep fighting.

No matter what, no matter how humiliating or painful things got, I always kept going. I think that's what made me stronger. I didn't want anything to defeat me or allow anyone to pity me, even during my most vulnerable moments. Despite this, I never saw that strength in myself or in all the things I did to survive because I was blindsided by my seizures. I often thought that I was weak, though I clearly wasn't. My thoughts were very negative most of the time, and that wore me down. It made me vulnerable to self-pity. After I finally became seizure free, I realized that when I was still living with seizures, whenever I felt depressed, helpless, angry, or embarrassed, I would do things that made me happy and that made me persevere. I didn't do this consciously; it was just a natural impulse. I had already found my happy place without realizing it.

There was really no time when I was completely "safe" during my epilepsy journey. No matter what I did, there was always a risk. The Department of Motor Vehicles (DMV) in Hickory, North Carolina, did not forbid me from driving and issued me a license at the age of sixteen. I could usually feel an aura coming on, so I was able to pull over until the seizure passed. I was comfortable knowing that I could at least control that much. In hindsight though, I shouldn't have been driving all those years. And my parents definitely didn't want me to drive. It was their worst nightmare.

When I moved to Qatar after graduating from the University of Miami, I had a driver and a car at my service anytime I wanted to go somewhere. But I was young and headstrong, and only when it came to driving was I ever selfish in any way. I wanted to live my life. I wanted to be "normal," like everyone else. Dr. Thomas and Dr. Patrick didn't oppose it, so why should I? Now, it seems obvious why I shouldn't have been driving, but it wasn't obvious to me at the time.

I had convinced myself that it was okay to drive since none of my doctors in the US had ever told me not to and it hadn't stopped me from getting a driver's license there. I

Chapter Ten

When I first moved to Qatar after university, I had just recently started taking Topamax. I became paranoid at times, though not often. Sometimes, people would look at me, and I'd become agitated and want to snap, "What are you looking at?" I overanalyzed everything, thinking people were talking about me. I had many outbursts. I'm not normally a rude person, but I was easily provoked during this period and couldn't control my behavior. Once, I even snapped at a waiter in a restaurant for no reason. Fortunately, this never happened with the hotel employees where I lived. I wouldn't be able to live with myself if I were perceived as rude and high-handed because that's the complete opposite of who I truly am. I was raised to be respectful to all, regardless of age, job, race, or religion. Being the RVPO's daughter, I was extraordinarily spoiled, but I was taught to treat everyone the same and with full respect and to never be materialistic or brag about my privileges. My parents taught me to be appreciative and to count my blessings. I'm so thankful for that upbringing, and I work very hard to make sure my two boys are raised the same way.

Sometimes, your medication will get the best of you. Your mind will play tricks on you. In my experience, the side effects of Topamax were horrible. It gave me severe brain fog, and I could feel the difference when the fog cleared. Some of these side effects destroyed parts of my life just as effectively as epilepsy did. The seizures themselves and the electrical discharges between the seizures can impair normal brain functions, contribute to behavioral problems, and might even create chemical imbalances in the brain that lead to psychiatric difficulties.

Therapy would have undeniably helped me. A therapist would have taught me how to shift my mindset through a technique called cognitive reframing. However, I didn't want to seek therapy back then. I was already living with epilepsy and felt like seeing a therapist as well was just too much. It seemed embarrassing, and I was afraid someone would find out. Plus, I was convinced that I was handling things on my own—though I definitely wasn't. I ignored my mental health instead of empowering it, and that's what was weighing me down. I see now that therapy would've saved me a lot of pain and suffering and also that there's no shame in seeking help. If I could go back in time and change one thing, it would definitely be to go to therapy.

One time, an awful incident happened while I was having a seizure. I was having dinner with Nadine and her fiancé Edward (Eddie) in a Mexican restaurant that also had music and a dance floor. The restaurant was in the hotel I was living in at the time. I was on the dance floor, just having fun, when I started to have a seizure. A guy came up behind me and thought I was drunk. Probably thinking that he could easily do whatever he wanted to me, he made a lewd and disgusting pass at me.

Luckily, Eddie, my now-brother-in-law, stepped in and had him kicked out for harassment. While I was grateful, I couldn't help but wonder, "What would have happened if Eddie wasn't there? What if things had gotten worse?" In such situations, things can go from bad to worse very quickly.

Afterward, the humiliation I felt was crippling. It led me to believe that the situation was somehow my fault and that I was partly to blame for what happened. People can be quick to judge you, but to be cruel like that is pure evil. An incident like this leaves a mark. In my case, it made me very cautious and self-protective, even in situations that most people would find normal.

Pain is invisible. You can't see it. I experienced so much pain that no one ever knew about, some of it in the form of self-harm. I would bang my right fist against the wall or even sharp objects—whatever was in front of me at the moment I'd breakdown—until my fist was purple and blue, sometimes bleeding. I didn't do it for attention. In fact, nobody knew. I only did this when I felt impossibly frustrated and angry, with no hope. When I got to that point, my mind would start to play games with me, trying to convince me that hurting myself more was the only or the best way to deal with my pain. I had so many questions but no answers. After I banged my fist until it bruised and started to come back to my senses, I would ask myself why I was doing this.

I really tried not to fall into self-pity. I didn't want my disorder and medications to cloud my judgment. But sometimes, at the end of the day, banging my fist felt like the only way to release all my complicated emotions. Self-harm was also a side effect of my medications, an uncontrollable impulse.

There were long-term consequences to my first banging. I stopped hurting myself after I became seizure free and went off the medications with the horrible side effects, but to this day, my right hand is extremely weak. I'm right-handed, so when I overuse it, I can feel the muscles and joints strain in my fingers, especially when I clench my fist to do things like open a sealed jar, writing too much, or gripping my squash racquet for too long. After my boys were born, my hand would sometimes jerk when they held it because even their gentle pressure was painful. Wearing rings on that hand back then was almost impossible. Even doing the dishes with cold water would hurt.

I'm very sad that I went this route because I used to get many compliments on my hands, even from strangers. Once, I was at a check-in counter at the airport in Jordan, and the lady behind the counter commented on how nice my hands looked. Another time, one of my advertising clients in Qatar, Ali Bin Ali Watches and Jewelers, asked me to do an advertisement for a magazine, using my hand to display jewelry. They covered my hand with thousands of dollars' worth of beautiful diamonds and took countless photos. Similarly, my hands appeared in an advertisement for a local brand of tissues in Jeddah, Saudi Arabia.

This self-harm behavior made me feel ashamed of myself. I am grateful for everything I have been blessed with, including my hands. In my normal state of mind, I would never want to harm myself like that. It was a mental impulse that was beyond my control. When I was in a better state of mind, I felt guilty for this behavior because I have so much love and support in my life, and it felt like I was betraying everyone who gave me their unconditional love and support. I didn't want them to feel like this wasn't enough, since it was truly more than enough.

This went on throughout the rest of my journey with epilepsy, and even though there are justifications for my actions, I always felt ashamed of it. A lifetime of taking such medications can have permanent side effects that become a part of who you are, and 90 percent of anti-epileptic medications share the same side effects. However, the worst phase of my life occurred while I was in Qatar while I was taking Topamax, and my paranoia completely vanished after I stopped taking Topamax. None of the other medications I took over the years had the side effect of paranoia and weight loss.

Topamax also caused awful mood swings. I could turn on someone in a heartbeat, going from being my usual kind self one moment to being very mean and oversensitive the next. People perceived me as rude and unfriendly. Unfortunately, not everyone had the empathy to understand that the real me was hidden behind my seizures and the powerful medications I was taking to control them. The drugs messed with my ability to interact socially. They screwed up my relationships with the people I loved and saw on a regular basis, like with my best friend Nisreen in Jordan and family members like my cousin Tarek's wife Soula, who was living in Qatar at the time. My mom, dad, and Nadine knew what I was going through, but not many others did. With the brain fog I experienced, it was sometimes hard for me to recognize myself, let alone try to explain to others what I was going through. People don't always get the whole story. I hated what I was going through and who I seemed to be becoming, but I didn't have any control over it.

Nisreen recalls how difficult my early adulthood was, due not only to my seizures but also to my mental health issues. She says of this period:

> Pre-marriage and teens, I have seen her have a lot of seizures. There was a phase where I didn't see seizures. There was a change in her. She was doubtful. She'd analyze things, and not in a positive way. That was the biggest change pre- and post-surgery I saw in her.

Chapter Eleven

My hardest, darkest days were in Qatar. I wish I hadn't lived through them, and I try so hard to block them out. But when they do cross my mind, I thank God that I'm in a better place and that I can now articulate my feelings. I make sure to focus on the silver lining of how far I've come since then.

Sadly, if Topamax had completely controlled my seizures, I would have gladly sacrificed my mental health, because nothing is worse than having a seizure. If this medication is working for you, stick with it. I understand the difficult choices you're facing, and I feel your pain and struggle. However, if you're taking Topamax, still having seizures, and suffering from terrible, overpowering side effects, ask your neurologist if you can try a different medication. It still might not control your seizures, but if Topamax isn't either, you'll be free of what it's doing to you.

Topamax did work for me at first. It reduced my seizures when I started taking it in the US, and I never considered changing it. I only stopped taking Topamax when I wanted to get pregnant and found out that it can be fatal to a fetus. So, I replaced it with Lamictal and stayed on

Depakene. If it weren't for my desire to have children, I probably would've continued taking Topamax much longer.

The combination of Lamictal and Depakene didn't change the frequency of my seizures, but my mental health recovered a great deal. The paranoia and weight loss I experienced while on Topamax evaporated. This was noticeable to me and to everyone around me. If I had known this would happen, I wouldn't have waited to make this change nor forced myself to endure all that mental suffering.

A couple years later, I replaced Depakene with Levetiracetam, the generic form of Keppra, while staying on Lamictal as well. With this new combination, the frequency of my seizures did decrease a little, but they didn't go away entirely. Clearly, none of these anti-epileptic drugs were working, even though I was always taking a combination of two medications. My seizures were drug-resistant, and my only hope for becoming seizure free was surgery.

If you are facing the same thing and feeling hopeless, look into having the surgery. I waited too long, so if you qualify as a candidate, don't wait. Go for it. It changed my life forever.

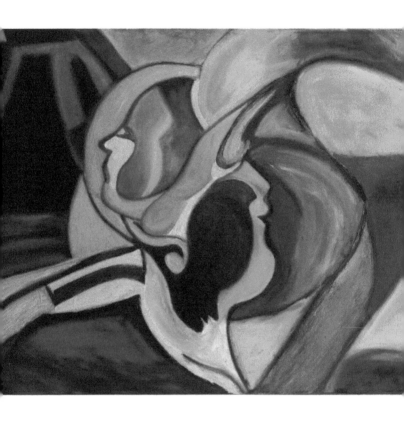

A Colorful Mind

Perfectly fine it all seems to be
you can never say out loud the anger you feel

It only destroys you and empowers your fears

Calling out for a hopeless plea will only echo to eternity
by the shade it casts let it burn endlessly

You will surrender to this life no matter what it takes
there's no way to change the bitter, it's a path that is forever
stained

Not running scared but desperate to push away the clouds
with a smile that struggles through tears, can't mend broken
blue skies

Drifting thoughts wither through a colorful mind
washing them away leads your mind to fantasize

Stop your whining, pretend everything is ok
that won't change a thing, the sky will remain cold and gray

It only makes you cry dry tears and makes you fall still

You will surrender to this life no matter what it takes
there's no way to change the bitter, it's a path that is forever
stained

talking. In fact, I talked so much that my friends occasionally got frustrated with me and teased me when I wouldn't let them get a word in.

My youngest cousin Samar first saw my angry, paranoid side during a visit while I was living in Qatar. We were in my yellow VW Beetle car, driving back home from somewhere. She was about twelve years old at the time and just happy to be hanging out. I was playing a song on the car stereo when she suddenly exclaimed, "Oh, I love this song!"

Out of nowhere, I snapped, "Oh, why? Because I told you earlier that it's my favorite song, so now, it has to be your favorite song, too?" It was so unlike me to be so rude and immature. To this day, I don't know how I could have been so cruel and pathetic. When I calmed down later, I felt like an impetuous fool. I had been paranoid and short-tempered and said hurtful things that I didn't mean and truly wished I could take back.

Samar was confused by my outburst. She was scared stiff, hurt, and didn't know why she was being attacked for no reason. The incident stuck with her for years. Later, when I got married and moved to Jerusalem, she was older and better able to understand and tolerate my mood swings and paranoia.

Another time, I was visiting Soula at the Arab Bank, where she worked. While we were in the reception area, I had the pleasure of meeting the bank manager, her boss. Soula briefly introduced us, and we chatted for a bit.

Later that day, Soula and Tarek came over to our house. Teasingly, Soula said, "Guess what my boss said about you after you left?"

Her thought-provoking question automatically pushed all my negative-thinking buttons. I was immediately on the defensive.

She then repeated the expression he'd used in Arabic, which meant that I am very clever.

He was giving me a compliment, but because my Arabic wasn't perfect, I misunderstood it and thought he was bad-mouthing me. Rather than simply asking her what the expression meant, I assumed the worst. I snapped at poor Soula, "How dare he say that about me? Who does he think he is? I'll put him in his place!"

Soula had witnessed these preposterous outbursts before, and she already knew this side of me. She accepted it because she knew who I really was. Why else would she have chosen me to be the godmother for her daughter, Anya? We laugh about this incident now, but when it happened, I was frantic with anger and unreasonable suspicion.

Another similar incident occurred while I was having dinner with Soula, Tarek, and my second cousin, Elias at a Chinese restaurant in Qatar. Everything was fine; we ordered our food and were having a nice time. As the waiter was bringing Soula her food, he accidentally bumped into my chair. Really, it was more like a gentle tap. The chair barely moved, and it could have easily gone unnoticed. Normally, I would've reacted sympathetically and told him not to worry about it. But instead, I lashed out at the guy. I got up, picked up my chair, thumped it on the ground, and said, "Here, are you happy now? You want me out of my chair? Couldn't you see that someone was sitting in it? At least have the decency to apologize." Some people might act this way naturally during mishaps, but not me. That isn't me, and it truly saddens me that I behaved that way. I couldn't even justify myself at the time because I wasn't in my right mind and didn't realize just how out of line I was.

These are just a few of my many humiliating moments. At such times, things would get foggy around me, and I

117

Chapter Fourteen

Navigating life with epilepsy with family and friends is complicated enough; dating just seemed like another thing to "deal with." Dimitri, however, was different. He really was my one and only. Here's how it happened.

Dimitri was good friends with my cousins Tarek and Samer, and we met through them as kids. Back then, we were just friends, but our relationship grew over time. My whole life, we frequently traveled to Jerusalem to visit my mom's family there, and my parents have an apartment in the same family-owned building they all live in. Dimitri lived nearby, and we saw each other all the time as kids, often riding our bikes or skateboards together. He was just always around. We remained friends as teenagers, and when I visited, we'd hang out.

During one of those visits, we went to a restaurant with a bunch of friends and my cousins. There was food, drinks, and a dance floor; it was a real party atmosphere. Dimitri asked me to dance, and it was obvious to everyone that we had lots of chemistry. We just clicked. Some of my friends made my long dress even longer. I'm sure I looked funny, holding up my long dress with one hand and carrying my heels with the other.

Despite this, it ended up being very romantic! We spent some time talking honestly about our feelings. He said that he wanted to propose to me but needed to clear away a few strings that were still attached. Of course, I took that to mean he needed to break up with someone else. We shared our first kiss that night.

He surprised me for Valentine's Day by coming to see me in Dubai. It's very difficult to get reservations in Dubai, especially during special occasions, because it's so commercialized there. He had to make the reservations weeks in advance, and he planned it all so well.

During dinner, he finally cleared up the misunderstanding about his supposed proposal to another girl. As it turned out, he was casually seeing another girl, but my cousins thought he was getting more serious than he really was. This story made its way through my family, and as with all games of telephone, by the time it reached me, it had morphed into a marriage proposal. Still, he decided not to deny the rumors; he hoped that the news would make me jealous and that I would finally admit how I felt about him. Clearly, it worked.

During his visit, he witnessed the terrible side of me that he had never seen before:

We were walking around at the mall when suddenly Janine started getting mad at me. I wasn't doing anything, at least I didn't think so. She said I was conspiring against her. She told me that I didn't love her. She just went off on me and then she took off. I didn't follow her because I didn't understand what was happening. I just turned around and went back to her house.

I told Aunt Norma about what had happened. It was very weird. I started packing to leave. I didn't know how to deal with it. I was completely in shock. I didn't know if I would go stay at a hotel or leave for the airport.

Aunt Norma explained to me that this was a side effect of the Topamax medication she was taking. Paranoia and anxiety could lead to such an incident, and paranoia and anxiety are side effects of Topamax.

Even though I grew to understand it later, this incident stuck with me for quite some time, and it was very difficult for me. At first, I wanted to leave. I wanted nothing to do with it until Aunt Norma explained what was going on. After that I read about the epilepsy medications and got more educated about all its side effects. I realized how difficult it must be for her to handle it because the real Janine I know, and love was nothing of the sort and that these side effects weren't going to get in the way of marrying her. In sickness and in health, in sorrow and in joy till death do us part.

We got engaged a few months later. When Dimitri came to propose to me, my dad said to him, "You do know Janine has an illness, right?"

Dimitri responded, "Yeah, and? It doesn't change the way I feel about her."

We got married one year later, on August 7, 2005.

Dimitri is very kind, caring, loving, and supportive. He's done so much for me and loves me unconditionally. He helps a lot with the boys and takes great care of us. He has sacrificed so much for me, yet never makes me feel like a burden. I will always be thankful for having such a blessing of a husband. He is always there for me, has gone to every single doctor's appointment with me, and has taken me to all my medical tests. He fights my

Chapter Sixteen

I knew that the only way to cope with my disorder and survive was to confront it with confidence, so that's exactly what I did. That was something I could control. I never allowed anyone to think less of me. In fact, some were even intimidated by me because I didn't give anyone the opportunity to pity me for my disorder.

Being a newlywed and moving to Jerusalem, away from my parents and Nadine, I was lucky to have so many family members around me. My aunts Salwa and Anisa are like second mothers. They are very special to me, and they have always taken such great care of me and my boys. They still give me the best advice when I need it, and they are my greatest comfort. My uncles Sameer, Maurice, and Nicolas and his wife, Aunt Hala, have always been there for me, too. I love them all more than they'll ever know, and I owe them so much for their endless love, care, and kindness. I would do anything for them.

My Aunt Salwa, who is also my Godmother was always very discreet in how she looked out for me:

Whenever Janine was around, I would always keep a close eye on her and make sure to sit in the direct line of sight of her to protect her without her being aware of it and to not make her feel uncomfortable. If I felt that something was wrong, I would quietly come near her and take her aside because I knew how she felt about not wanting to be the center of attention during a seizure even if she was with just family who already knew about it. If I were to be mistaken, then I would act like I was coming to ask her something. There was a time we were having lunch at my brother Nicolas's house with everyone else in the building when I saw her looking a bit off. I quietly got up off my chair and came beside her. I tried to be inconspicuous, I was very calm and acted like I needed to ask her something in the kitchen. We both walked together to the kitchen, and she suddenly held my hand and said to me say something nice and I said I love you and just like that it was over. I was so relieved that it went completely unnoticed, both because it was short and that I was able to spare her from being asked if she was okay by everyone afterward. We both know it's out of love and concern that they do that, but I knew how she felt about that. When I heard that she decided to have the surgery, I was terrified. I remember her talking about it a long time ago and I was so relieved back then when she said it wasn't an option. Now, it was really happening, and I made sure she wouldn't know how I felt because I saw how ready she was. She's always been and still is a very courageous girl.

My Aunt Anisa was present the day I had that very high fever and convulsions as a baby. She was the one who put me in the tub before rushing me to the pediatrician. She recalls:

I remember the day Janine had her first convulsions when she was a baby and we rushed her to the hospital. At that time, we didn't understand why the convulsions were happening. When she got older, I was in shock when I heard about her seizures. How could this have happened and what was the reason for it? When we all learned that the cause of her epilepsy was due to that high fever she had when she was a baby, it left me thinking that maybe the doctor back then could've given her some sort of medication after hearing about her high fever leading to convulsions. This may have helped her and not affected her in the future. I always made sure to keep a close eye on her so that if she was to have a seizure, I would be close by to help her. If I saw her staring with glassy eyes and moving her hands, I would run right over. My husband Maurice and I used to travel with her and her children to Dubai just in case something were to happen, we'd be with her and to make sure they'd arrive safely. There were a few episodes that really affected me, one was when she was walking out of the grocery shop while I was waiting in the car and she suddenly stopped and I saw that her lips were moving, it took me a second to realize that she was having a seizure and by the time I got to her, the seizure had passed. Another time was while I was with her in the car. She was driving, and everything was ok, but then she pulled over on the side of the road. I asked her why she stopped and then I noticed that she was about to have a seizure. There was also the time at Salwa's house where she had a very bad seizure, we were all panicking, and Samar fainted. That one was unforgettable. When she decided to do the surgery, I refused this idea, I was outraged. I didn't tell her at that time, but I told Norma and Johnny that she shouldn't do it and continuing to *have seizures is better than risk losing her memory or maybe worse. I felt a strong apprehension as to how her parents, Nadine and Dimitri agreed to this, I couldn't understand it and now I thank God for the success of her surgery and that she's completely healed and free to do anything she wants. She's a very special person, not only to me but to the whole family.*

The splendor of family doesn't stop with mine. Dimitri's family has always been very good to me, too, even before they knew me well. When Dimitri told his mom that he wanted to propose to me, he said, "Listen, I know Janine has an illness, but I love her. Uncle Johnny told me that there are many things I needed to know, and I'm okay with it."

She said, "It's okay. There's nothing wrong with someone having a medical condition. As long as you love her and she loves you, the rest will be fine."

Aunt Antoinette and Uncle Yousef were completely accepting of me from the start. They both knew my parents because they all grew up in Jerusalem, but still, they could've had reservations about me. But they never did, nor did Dima or Edgar. I love them for accepting me for who I am, for not judging me by my disorder, and for letting my unintentional behavior go unnoticed. They gave me my space, tolerated me, supported me, and never interfered in my personal life. I am deeply grateful and blessed to be loved by them all. Dima gave me the honor of being the godmother to her youngest son, George and to her daughter, Grace, at her first communion.

Aunt Antoinette did tell me over the years that it used to break her heart when Joseph and Johnny would cuddle me when I had a seizure. She still marvels at how brave they have always been about my epilepsy.

When I first moved to Jerusalem, Dimitri and I were invited to a dinner party. I already knew most of his friends from the many visits I'd made before getting married, but I didn't know there would be so many people there. At one point that evening, Soula asked me if I would mind talking to a mother and her teenage daughter who suffered from seizures. The girl's mother didn't know much about epilepsy and felt helpless as to how to help her daughter, Rinal, because she didn't understand what she was going through.

Rinal's mom wasn't alone in this. It's extremely difficult to know what's happening within a person who is battling epilepsy or to understand how much their seizures and medication can affect their mindset in daily life. Without a moment of hesitation, I agreed. Rinal's mother and I talked for quite a while.

During the car ride home, I kept thinking about our conversation and whether I had given Rinal and her mom any hope.

From that day on, I occasionally called Rinal or met her for coffee so she could talk with someone who understood her experiences, even though she was much younger than me. I shared a few of my stories and answered any questions she had. I wanted her to know that everything she was facing was normal and that she wasn't alone. I explained to her that no matter how much she tries to justify herself to others, they will never understand what she's going through. From what she told me, it was obvious that she was also suffering from epilepsy medication side effects, though she didn't realize it; the medication was behind many of her troubles.

The things she described were all too familiar to me. When I was her age, I never considered opening the leaflet that came inside the medication box and reading about the

Chapter Seventeen

First comes love, then comes marriage, then comes... you know the rest. Of course, Dimitri and I wanted children, but that was yet another challenge to navigate with epilepsy. Everything had to be carefully considered and planned—even more than if we were a typical married couple.

When we decided to have children, I was still on Topamax and Depakene. I went to a gynecologist who told me that Topamax carries a high risk of causing birth defects, including fatal harm. If I wanted to safely have children, I would need to replace the Topamax with a different medication. This wouldn't happen overnight. I had to gradually wean myself off the Topamax to minimize the potential for increased seizure frequency.

During both my pregnancies, I took regular dosages of two types of anti-epileptic medication, Lamictal and Depakene. Dr. Mark, the neurologist I was seeing at the time, didn't think I needed to increase my medication dosage. However, in 2014, during a visit with a senior neurologist in Dubai, he told me that he increased the medication dosage

I screamed my lungs out to my mom and dad; "Janine is not coming back, come quickly!" The thoughts running in my head, her eyes turning white, flipping backwards, that never happened except once in front of me, when I was five years old. I tried hard to recall what to do in that case, but my body froze, as hers froze as well.

My mother came rushing, dad told her to hold Janine's tongue so she wouldn't bite it, and he hurried to get a spoon to keep the tongue in place. I was never the coward, but at that moment, I was frozen, time itself froze for me. My father pushed me outside the kitchen and screamed, "Call the ambulance."

I backed out slowly into the corridor opposite the kitchen; my eyes still on her, on those blood stains from when she unconsciously bit on my mother's fingers that were holding her tongue. I look at her, and at her belly; there's Joseph inside, her first-born-to-be, my first nephew-to-be (though I had other nephews and nieces in Jerusalem, but Joseph was way too special for me). All I could hear was my cousins' rushing thumping on the stairs and around me, and all I could see was her, and her very pregnant belly. My eyes went dark, and in my thoughts was one constant sentence playing on repeat: "Please don't let her slip away from me." It was all dark, I didn't know if I lost her, or lost my own consciousness.

I was awakened minutes later by one of my cousins, or maybe it was my father. I was laying on the corridor floor. "Samar, wake up, wake up, Janine is okay." But I couldn't make out what was happening, why was I on the floor, and where was Janine?

As I gained consciousness, I rushed into my parents' bedroom, where she was somewhat sleeping, tired from what happened, and two paramedics were in the room ready to take her to the hospital.

I rarely like to recall that night, because despite the tens of times I witnessed Janine's seizures, that was the only night I ever felt hopeless, helpless, and I disappointed myself. I wasn't able to let it pass, no matter how much I told her I loved her, at that point in that night, "love" wasn't enough.

It's silly, but since that night I guess I started telling her I love her more, regardless, whether she was going through a seizure or not, it was my "just in case" way of making sure she's always there, and my own affirmation that I'll always be there.

When I woke up, I was lying on my aunt's bed with the paramedics by my side. I told them that I didn't need to go to the hospital because I was fine. The seizure was over. Why go to the hospital if there was nothing they could do? But as always, it was hospital policy that they take me. I was also quite pregnant, which was another concern.

When I reached the hospital, the nurse wasn't sensitive to my condition. She applied too much pressure while doing my internal sonogram, with no consideration for the pain she was causing me. I was discharged several hours later in the exact same state I'd been in when I arrived. If only the paramedics had listened to me and not taken me to the emergency room, I could at least have rested and recovered at home.

Seizures wouldn't leave me alone, even after giving birth.

When I gave birth to Joseph, my mom was with me. My water broke at 8 a.m., and he was born at 11:47 p.m. on July 24, 2007. It was a very tough birth; I was gritting my teeth so hard the entire time. Then, I had a grand mal seizure about an hour after delivery and another one while I was asleep. Still, all that mattered was that he was born healthy.

during a seizure she had him welded in her arms. How strong a mother's intuition is.

I can't begin to describe the horror I felt when I came out of that seizure. Holding Joseph in my arms, not knowing what could've happened, I was terrified.

After that, Dimitri and my parents thought it would be best to get a full-time nanny from abroad to be with me and help me during the day while Dimitri was at work. Bringing someone from abroad as domestic help is very restricted in Israel, and you have to have a very high level of disability. Even though my situation was desperate, I didn't qualify. I would have to get by on my own, relying on friends and family to help.

Finding someone local to help around the house on a daily basis is impossible; you're lucky to find someone who'll come for a few hours once a week. People here are always looking for someone to help around the house, and if they're lucky, they'll find someone through word of mouth. That's how I found Maha. She had been working at my aunt's house for years, going there three times a week. When I first got married and moved to Jerusalem, they gave up one of their days so she could come and help me once a week.

When Joseph was about one year old, he developed a high fever of 40 degrees Celsius (104 Fahrenheit). I was very worried and rushed him to the clinic. I was terrified, trying to hold back my tears. After all, I developed epilepsy as a result of a high fever as a baby. Now, I was bringing my baby into the clinic with a high fever.

After I checked him in at the clinic, I had to go to the nurse's station so she could take his temperature. By then, his fever had gone down a bit because I had given him some medicine earlier that helped reduce it.

Heading toward the pediatrician's office, I saw that two ladies and their children were ahead of me, waiting to see the doctor. When I got there, I purposely stood with my back toward them, facing the wall while holding Joseph in my arms. I couldn't hold back my tears any longer, so I tried to hide them by tilting my face to the side and wiping them on my shoulder. There was no other way to get rid of them because I was holding Joseph in my arms.

Despite my best efforts, it was obvious that I was crying. One of the two ladies, whose turn was next, came up to me, tapped me on the shoulder, and asked if I was okay. I said I was, but she could tell I wasn't. She offered to let me go in ahead of her, which was very kind of her.

When I entered the pediatrician's office, he was confused as to why I was wiping away tears. He said, "I see that Joseph has a fever, but why are you crying? Mothers are so affectionate toward their children! I can tell that he's your firstborn."

I told him that I was worried because my epilepsy developed as a result of a high fever I had when I was a baby. He explained that epilepsy is a result of a rapid jump in temperature, which leads to convulsions, not just a high fever. For years, I had worried that any high fever in babies would cause epilepsy. I was relieved to learn that that wasn't the case.

Pregnancy wasn't much easier the second time around.

February 14, 2009, was Uncle Samir's birthday, and everyone was celebrating at his apartment, which is one floor below my parents' apartment. I was pregnant with my youngest son, Johnny Junior, and was feeling a bit tired. So, I left and went upstairs to my parents' place. Just like when I was pregnant with Joseph, I had a grand mal seizure, only this time, I was alone. Fortunately, a mother's intuition led my mom to come up and see what I was

My first tattoo featured Joseph's and Johnny's names in an infinity symbol. It's a very common tattoo, but it's very meaningful to me. My boys are the sun in my sky. They are my world.

October and November brings the olive harvest in Palestine, which is symbolic of our culture and traditions. Every year, my son's school takes its elementary students olive picking in groves owned by Palestinian families. One time, I volunteered to help with the olive brining activity for Joseph's class, as I had previously with Johnny's class. This involves the students gently smashing the olives they'd already picked with a stone and putting them in jars to brine.

While waiting outside the classroom for Joseph's lesson to finish, I had a seizure in the hallway. It wasn't a long one, but it caused me to look like I was aimlessly wandering the halls for a short time. A thirteen- or fourteen-year-old girl saw the whole thing. When I came out of my seizure, I found myself far from the classroom on the opposite side of the hallway, and she was standing in front of me, looking as confused as I was. She was panicky and repeatedly asked me if I was okay. I assured her that I was, and she took off, still puzzled. Moments later, when I entered the classroom, Joseph's teacher noticed that I wasn't myself and asked if there was anything wrong. I told her what had happened, just in case I had another seizure. She asked if I'd like to go home and rest, but that's not usually necessary after a complex-partial seizure. So, I stayed and enjoyed working with Joseph and his classmates.

Still, this incident caused a great deal of internal conflict for me. Teenagers often gossip about things they've seen and tend to unintentionally exaggerate. I'm sure this girl told her friends and family about what happened that day at school. And who wouldn't? After all, it's not something you see every day. I could easily see myself becoming the talk of students. How would my boys feel if that girl happened to know who I was or was later able to point me out? I couldn't remember her face because I was unconscious during my seizure and confused after it, so I wouldn't be able to find her to explain what had happened and ask her to keep quiet about it—not for my sake, but for the sake of my boys. They were both fairly popular with a lot of friends, but what would gossip about me do to them? Would kids start to bully them or talk about them behind their backs? What if she had a smartphone and recorded me having a seizure? What if, what if, what if... These are the kinds of thoughts that ran through my mind as a mother who also happened to have seizures. Not only was I worried about the seizure itself, but also, I was worried about my boys and what gossip about it would do to them. This led back to familiar thoughts: "How are they handling their mother having this disorder? What is it doing to their lives? This is so unfair to them..." You can see how quickly and easily my thoughts started to twirl downward.

I also can't begin to imagine what it was like for Dimitri all those years. How he managed to live with all this—the challenges, the fear, the sacrifice, the constant worrying, always having to take care of me when I had a seizure—is beyond me. He's an amazing and very supportive husband and is just as much a fighter as me.

Six years after my surgery, I got another tattoo, this one of a purple epilepsy awareness ribbon and the word 'Fighter' below it. While awareness ribbons don't change the challenging reality of having epilepsy, they do serve as symbols of hope. But why the word 'Fighter,' rather than 'Survivor'? Because 'Survivor' means that you've survived and that the journey has ended. 'Fighter' means you will continue to support others still going through their own

By now, it was obvious that she was intentionally provoking me, so I threw a fit. Even leaving aside my medically induced temper, I was furious, and I wasn't going to stay silent just because there was a machine gun strapped to her side. My mom tried to calm me down because she was worried things would get out of hand, but I wouldn't listen.

My hands were excessively shaking with anger, but the soldiers now suspected that I was nervous because I was planning on doing something wrong. Shaking is another side effect of anti-epileptic medication. They surrounded me, then took me to the head of security, and he interrogated me. After that, I was taken into a room where I was strip-searched. This was very intimidating and humiliating, which only made things worse. In the end, I was detained for over two hours.

Growing up with very generous parents taught me a lot. They often quoted an Arabic proverb: "Do good and throw it in the sea." It means you should do something good for the sake of doing it, not because you expect something in return. During my engagement, when I was still living in Dubai with my parents, I selected five of my photographs of Jerusalem, printed one thousand digital copies of each in A4 size, and sold them for charity. I sold them at a very affordable price; a set of five in a big brown envelope sold for fifteen dollars. People from all parts of the world bought them, and some chose to overpay in support of the cause. My cousin Narmine's daughter, Joumana, took some and sold them at her school bazaar in Jordan. I'll never forget Uncle Jamil Wafa's generous donation of $1500 for a set of five. He is a close family friend who was a big part of my childhood.

Altogether, I raised a total of $20,000, more than I ever expected. I gave $15,000 to the Four Homes of Mercy, a nonprofit organization in Jerusalem that offers short-term, long-term, and respite care, including rehabilitation services, for children beginning at age four, all the way through old age. I donated the other $5,000 to Rawdat El Zuhur School in Jerusalem, another non-profit organization, who needed to install a central heating system because the students were freezing in class during the winter.

I wanted to do a good deed because I felt for those who were suffering. Even though I grew up with this difficult disorder and it wasn't pleasant for me, I always reminded myself that I still had it much better than others. This taught me to appreciate life and count my blessings every single day.

I have loved art ever since I was young, but I only started painting in 2010 after Johnny was born and I made the decision to stop driving. I had postpartum depression with Johnny, which made the side effects from my medications even worse. My attitude changed; I was more aggressive. It was very noticeable to family and friends, but they continued to accept me and didn't judge me.

Chapter Twenty-One

When I first got married and moved to Jerusalem from Dubai, I decided to start driving again. You would think I'd learned my lesson from my first accident, but I couldn't bear the thought of having to be reliant on others. I was a newlywed settling into a new country, and I wasn't going to start off by feeling helpless. So, I bought a car and put my faith in God's hands. I avoided driving on days when I was at an increased risk of having a seizure. The seizure logs I had been keeping since I was first diagnosed with epilepsy revealed over time that my grand mal seizures tended to happen within a few days of my period. There was still the occasional surprise seizure, but they were generally brief. This system worked well for my first few years in Jerusalem. But then, one fine morning, that changed.

Dimitri was standing outside on the balcony, having a cigarette. He watched me drive out of our garage and away from the house. Then, when I was about two hundred meters down the road, he saw my car swerve toward the tree beside the road. He knew I was having a seizure, and he was right.

He came charging down two flights of stairs and sprinted the two-hundred-meter distance to the car. All he could see was that I was having a seizure. He didn't know that it was a short one and that I had already regained control while he was still running toward me. It was a thirty-second seizure, and I was driving at a very low speed when it happened. Still, I knew then that I wouldn't be driving anymore. It was only thanks to God's protection that something more serious didn't happen.

After that, I put my keys down and my car up for sale. It was a huge relief, both to me and to everyone around me. They wouldn't admit it, but they were always very concerned about my safety. I still had my license and could have kept driving, but I made the decision to stop of my own accord. Honestly, I shouldn't have been driving in the first place, and I was finally ready to accept that. Still, as anticipated, I lost all my independence when I stopped driving. I felt handicapped and incredibly depressed.

In February of 2016, four months after my surgery, the Road and Safety Department in Jerusalem came after me. It's standard procedure for hospitals to inform them when a person has brain surgery, since that person could now be a safety hazard on the road. I received a letter from them, saying my license was suspended. I had to go to their office and physically give them my license. They didn't know that I hadn't been driving for six years.

In reality, I can think of far worse things happening than having my license taken away, but at that moment, it felt like a slap in the face. When I gave it to the lady at the DMV office, she said, "Don't worry, it's only temporary. You'll get it back." In September of 2017, a year and a half after my surgery, I finally got my license back. Altogether, I was unable to drive for seven and a half years straight.

My friends and family knew how difficult it was for me

to be unable to drive all those years, but they made it a point to help me believe otherwise. Every time the subject of driving came up in conversation, there was a rush to point out how it's not the end of the world if one doesn't drive or to say that they wished they didn't have to drive and could have someone drive them around. I knew it was their way of trying to make me feel better. But regardless of how hard they tried to convince me that not driving wasn't a big deal, it didn't change how I felt.

I turned back to sports to help with my depression. I was very into sports as a kid. At first, I played squash alone. I couldn't find a partner in Jerusalem because I prefer to speak English and most of the people living near me spoke Arabic. My Arabic is fine; I just prefer English. Mostly, I also didn't want to put up with the stigma that came with my epilepsy. I'm sure I looked funny chasing the ball from side to side all alone, but it was a good way to get my anger and rage out. I did that for about five months.

While I lived in Dubai, Lara, a good friend of mine whom I met in Qatar and who had also moved to Dubai, was my squash partner. We would play together at least twice a week, and she kindly picked me up and dropped me back at home before and after our games, since I had stopped driving after my car accident in Qatar. Even while on vacation in Jordan, I would play squash with my cousin Runa.

In order to not feel imprisoned and handicapped by having to depend on others for rides, I started walking, rain or shine, when I needed to get things done. My family constantly worried about me having a seizure while walking down the street, but they understood why I did this. I did occasionally have seizures while I was out, but I got through them, and most of the time, I didn't tell anyone about them. Doing so would only make them worry and give them another reason to convince me to stop walking alone.

I can't say that I wasn't worried myself because I was, so I took extra precautions to feel safer. I would walk on the inside edge of the sidewalk, farthest away from the road. That way, if I had a seizure and fell down, I wouldn't get run over by a car. I mostly kept to the quieter neighborhoods, where there weren't too many cars driving by or people walking around.

One day, I had a complex-partial seizure while I was out walking and there was no one around. I got out of the seizure by mumbling words of prayer. I have so much faith in God that my subconscious mind would reach out to Him to save me and make the seizure stop when I was alone.

After that, I realized that I would be putting myself in great danger if I were to have a grand mal seizure when no one was around to help me—or, even worse, if I were to have a seizure and someone wanted to harm me while I was unconscious and helpless. So, despite how calm and peaceful my preferred walking routes were, I switched to walking through a much more crowded area, just to be on the safe side. I always found ways to not let my seizures control me. I did everything I put my mind to. I found solutions and made things happen.

Every other day, I would walk a total of about five kilometers to the nearest mall, just to grab a coffee and sometimes buy paint or get things for my boys. Then, I'd walk back home or go visit my aunts. Sometimes, I ended up carrying heavy shopping bags, but I wanted to feel free, to breathe, to lift my spirits, to not have to wait on others, and to not feel handicapped.

One time, I had a seizure while walking around the mall. I felt an aura coming on, so I quickly made my way to the nearest wall, hoping to stand beside it until the seizure

170

went away. As soon as I got there, my seizure started. When it was over, I found two much older Israeli women helping me. Their English was better than my Hebrew, and they asked if I was okay, if there was someone with me at the mall, or if they should call someone to come get me. I told them that I was fine, thanked them for their help, and went on my way.

Once a complex-partial seizure passes, everything goes back to normal within seconds. If it had been a grand mal seizure, things would've been much worse; I'd feel confused and tired and would need someone to come get me. I'm so glad that it wasn't a grand mal seizure. It wouldn't have stopped me from continuing my routine, but it would have caused a scene—maybe even a commotion—and I'd end up having to deal with the whole ambulance drill all over again.

Soon after that incident, I started going to the gym twice a week just to swim and blow off steam. I would go swimming one day and walk the next day. I started by swimming twenty laps and gradually worked up to one hundred laps in an hour and a half.

I've always loved to swim. I swam five hundred laps for a charity event at the age of twelve when I lived in Bahrain, coming in first place. I also came in second place at a charity bikeathon event in Bahrain.

Taxis aren't reliable in Jerusalem; they're usually five to ten minutes late. After swimming, I often found myself waiting in the street with wet hair, which was unpleasant in the winter. I couldn't wait inside, because the gym entrance is far from the street, so I wouldn't be able to see them. Even if I could, they look like regular civilian cars so I can't be sure it's them. Back then, the taxis didn't call to tell you they've arrived, they expect you to be waiting outside according to the time of arrival they'd given you. On the other hand, I also didn't want to risk having a seizure, because being cold is a trigger for me.

After having a seizure in the shower of the gym's changing room, I stopped showering at the gym. I was incredibly embarrassed, but it could have been much worse. I could have fallen in the shower, hit my head, gotten a concussion, and maybe swallowed a gallon of water before someone found me.

This didn't stop me from continuing my weekly routine, but I did start taking extra precautions, such as no longer showering at the gym, which was no big deal. I could do without, and it wasn't going to stop me from doing what I enjoyed and what was helping me release my frustrations. I always told myself, "I can, and I will." And in this case, I did.

Still, humiliating moments like these caught up with me on days when I was already feeling depressed, and I would dwell on them. There's no value in dwelling, but I'd end up being under a gray cloud that's hovering over me and following me around all the time and it's so difficult to escape it.

Chapter Twenty-Two

After I became seizure free, I stopped walking to the mall just to get out, but I continued to play sports. The boys and I participated in the Palestine Marathon in Bethlehem, organized by the Right to Movement running group. The race seeks to create international awareness about how Israeli occupation prevents Palestinian freedom of movement, which is a universally recognized human right. I also went back to playing squash a few years after that. One time on our car ride home I was telling Dimitri that I was planning on going back to playing squash on my own until I can find a partner. Joseph, fifteen years old at the time, interrupts and says, "teach me and I'll play with you." I thought he was joking, but later he kept on asking me when I was going to book the squash court so we can go play together. So, I went out and bought him a squash racquet, taught him the basic rules of the game and off we went to play together. After we were done practicing on our first day, a member from the club, watching us play, asked if Joseph would like to sign up for an upcoming squash training course seeing that he was keen on learning. It was the perfect opportunity for him to learn the sport with a

own dark thoughts. I'd try to figure things out, but I couldn't because I don't remember anything that happens during my seizures. I often played music at full blast in the car back when I was still driving just to silence the screams in my head.

Part of the problem was that Nadine and my parents lived so far away. I didn't want to worry them, but it was difficult to fool them. I didn't want to turn to alcohol because I knew I'd end up relying on it as a coping mechanism to numb my pain. I tried that while living in Qatar, and it didn't work. It was a temporary fix for something that couldn't be fixed. It wasn't worth ruining my reputation for such a fleeting relief. Instead, I turned to poetry and art, which says a lot about how I felt.

After I stopped driving, I could no longer take Joseph and my God daughter, Anya, to school. Dropping them off now became Dimitri's responsibility. Since he was still at work when it was time to pick them up, my Uncle Maurice and I would go get them together, since Anya was his granddaughter. By the time Johnny was old enough to go to nursery school, Joseph and Anya were attending the Jerusalem American School (JAS) kindergarten. So, the morning drop-off and afternoon pickup routine stayed the same, with the addition of a second school in the complete opposite direction.

When Dimitri started working in Ramallah, he had to leave home early each morning, which changed our routine. He took the boys to JAS and dropped them off around 7:15 a.m., which was very early, since school didn't start until 8 a.m.

One day, Tarek heard how early the boys were getting to school. Without a moment's hesitation, he said, "I didn't know they went to school so early! It's too cold for them to wait in the playground. From now on, why doesn't Soula pick them up on her way to school with the girls around 7:40? She passes along your road, so it's on her way."

It was so kind and thoughtful of him to offer and to empathize with the boys. I'm forever grateful to them both. They were living in the same building as my parents' apartment at the time, so they were very close by. After that, Soula would call me each morning a few minutes before she left home, and the boys and I would wait for her across the street so they could easily hop in the car quickly to avoid impatient drivers.

A couple of years later, a huge supermarket opened near our house, closing off the route Soula took to pick them up. That's when the boys finally started taking the bus to and from school. For years, everyone wanted to make sure the boys had options to get to school beyond the bus so I wouldn't feel more guilty than I already did as a parent, and I was very grateful. However, when they started taking the bus, I found that I was relieved. Things became less complicated for everyone, and it made me feel like less of a burden, though no one ever made me feel that way.

Allison and I met at Sunshine Nursery School, which both Joseph and her daughter, Maria, attended when they were young. We were allowed to be in class with them during their first week of school. Every day, we would reduce our time with the children by one hour and wait outside in the playground, just in case they needed us. By the end of that week, they were used to being on their own in school. During that week, Allison and I spent hours talking on the playground, and we just clicked. Our friendship quickly evolved, and we became good friends. We often took Maria and Joseph to activities together and had coffee while waiting for them. After I stopped driving, she drove us for these outings, and she never made me feel like a burden. She was a very good friend and a godsend. I will

There were a few times when Tarek and Soula took two cars just to fit me and the boys when Dimitri was working late which was very kind of them.

For many years during Christmas and summer vacations, the boys and I stayed with my parents in Dubai. Because Dimitri couldn't take much time off work, he wanted the rest of us to spend quality time with my parents and to fully enjoy our summer vacation. My Aunt Anisa—who is my mom's sister—and Uncle Maurice were kind enough to always travel with me and spend a couple of weeks at my parents' house. Then, Dimitri would come spend a few weeks with us when he could and travel back home with me and the boys. Then, in August, we would meet up somewhere else with Mom, Dad, Nadine, and her family for our yearly family reunion. When Dimitri started running his own business from home, he could be more flexible with travel plans, and he would spend the whole summer with us.

As much as I wanted to travel alone, it was never an option for me. Traveling alone was just too big a risk.

Chapter Twenty-Three

Dimitri must really love me. After all, he once risked arrest for me.

In the summer of 2015, a few months before my surgery, we were traveling to New York for our yearly family reunion with my parents, Nadine, and her family. On our return flight home, I had two grand mal seizures, one on the plane and one at the airport after landing.

Dimitri recalls:

During a flight home from the states, Joseph and I were sitting on one side of the plane, and Janine and Johnny on the other side. I spotted her having a grand mal seizure. I told Joseph not to move out of his seat, quickly unfastened my seatbelt and rushed over to help her. Johnny was scared and had already started panicking. I knew not to put my fingers in her mouth, but you want to try and control her tongue somehow, so I put a small plastic bottle of water in her mouth. Whatever I could find that wouldn't be dangerous to put in her mouth and luckily, I saw the empty plastic bottle in the pocket in front of her seat.

At the time it happened, the plane had just started its descent and the pilot had switched on the fasten seatbelt sign in preparation for landing. The flight attendant was furious and instructed me to sit down, but I was too focused on Janine and trying to control her seizure. On the flight intercom she started raising her voice and ordering me to sit down. I wasn't listening to her, so she must've thought I was ignoring her, and I could hear people around me muttering. She then threatened to have me arrested when the plane landed if I wouldn't sit down. Still not paying any attention to her, she said, "Sir, there will be two police officers ready to escort you off the plane upon arrival into Queen Alia International Airport. You have been warned too many times and failed to abide by the rules and will be held accountable." I finally came to my senses and yelled out my wife is having a seizure; she can hardly breathe. She rushed over to help me and brought an emergency oxygen mask tank with her, while the other flight attendant gave a cabin announcement asking if there was a doctor or nurse on board to please come forward. A nurse on the flight came over and started helping me. Her seizure finally came to an end as we were landing. It's one of those seizures I don't like to recall because I felt as if I was losing her. The boys were so worried and crying, frightened for their mom. This seizure would've required an ambulance. Well, what do you know when you need one, it's nowhere to be found. That is why Janine doesn't travel alone and why she always must have someone with her.

We always sit together on the plane, as any family would do. To guarantee that we'll sit together on long distance flights, Janine would pay in advance to reserve the seats if given the option by the airline upon purchasing our tickets. Unfortunately, that wasn't an option on this flight and the flight was full.

On that same trip, we landed in Jordan, and we were going to take a connecting flight to Tel Aviv. The boys and Janine hadn't eaten on the plane, so I sat them down and I got their orders for food. I left them to go get the food in a food court type setting. I always tried to keep them in my direct line of sight, even if I had to walk away from them. This time, I couldn't see them, because there was a wall between us. I wasn't too worried though, because Janine had already suffered a very bad seizure on the plane and usually when she has an attack like that, you would never expect a second one to follow, at least not another strong one.

I was working on getting the food, when suddenly I heard a commotion and I saw people staring in the direction where I knew Janine and the boys were. I knew something was wrong, so I took off running. I even knocked a couple of people over to get to her. Janine was having another seizure, as strong as the one on the plane. I remember trying to get people out of the way so I could get to her. I was cursing and shouting at people, and I even pushed one guy away. I could have gotten my ass kicked. But I was scared. It's normal for people to gather around to see what's happening and why the sudden commotion, but I needed to get there because most people don't know what to do and especially during a strong grand mal seizure, not knowing what to do can be life threatening. I finally got to them.

After that was all over, Janine calmed down, and I hugged her and the boys. It was a very emotional moment.

Living with someone with epilepsy is a special kind of life that needs special attention. It requires sacrifices. It requires rational thinking because you have to find solutions. My professional background is in private equity investments. We buy failing companies. We flip them, make them profitable then sell them. In this process there are no emotions.

You think about reaching the goal. If that means firing 100 people, so be it. It's not the time to be emotional. You must think in this same rational way with epilepsy. You can't think with your heart. The first thing you have to do is figure out how to get rid of it. Do your research, learn what you need to learn, and then make the best decision you can with your head, not your heart.

In Janine's situation, I was pushing for her surgery when a lot of people around her were against it. I wanted her to do it in 2012, long before she actually did. Why?

She was getting worse and worse. Medications weren't helping her health any longer. And the problem also was, as she got older, would the medications work differently, or not work at all? And what if, by then, it was too late to do the surgery? There comes a point when you have to cut your losses. You have to take risks. For me, the end was clear. She was only going to get worse, until she does the surgery.

I was all for the surgery in spite of the risks and in spite of how many people were against it. I did research, checked out how much equipment and technology have improved. I checked doctors' success rates. I was taking logical steps. I was used to doing Risk/Benefit analyses for my work. I did the same thing when considering the surgery.

For a while, I was alone in my desire to have Janine get the surgery. That was all about to change.

For years, I consulted numerous neurologists and

specialists all over the world, whether in person, over the phone, or via email. My parents continuously sought out the best specialists in the field and advocated that I get second and third opinions on everything. Our shared aim was finding a cure for my seizures.

In addition to traditional medication, I tried various alternative medicine techniques, such as acupuncture, Reiki, and attunement therapy.

I did a lot of work with Reiki. In the summer of 2001, I met Levon through my Uncle Maurice. He insisted that I call Levon because he sincerely believed he could help me with my seizures. My dad called him one afternoon on my behalf—I felt that it would be easier for my dad to talk to him than me, since my uncle was the one who knew Levon —and explained my problem. Levon assured him that he would try to help reduce the frequency of my seizures and possibly cure them. During that same phone call, he requested some personal information about me, such as my full name, mother's maiden name, date of birth, time of birth, and horoscope. He said I should visit him in a couple of days to review my personal information.

A few days later, I went to meet Levon in person. I gave him a brief summary of my life, and he asked me a couple of questions. Then, he explained what he did.

He had already prepared a mixture of seven different natural herbs, plus a mixture of different oils. He instructed me to drink the herbs with boiled water every day at specific times. After I finished drinking it, I should pour the remaining herb bits over plants rooted in the soil, as he had prayed over the herbs, and they were therefore sacred. He also gave me a small, sealed sachet with a tiny sliver of wood from a cross and other religious items and advised me to always keep them in my possession for protection and good luck. Finally, he told me to look at the full moon every time it was in the sky and to then turn and look at something green. He refused any payment; all he asked was that I light a tall candle in the Holy Sepulchre Church in Jerusalem when I became seizure free, which I eventually did.

Reiki means 'universal life energy.' It is a hands-on healing technique that uses a person's life force energy to balance their body physically, emotionally, mentally, and spiritually. During a Reiki session, the people involved must remove all metal items from their bodies, as metal can interfere with the energy forces. Reiki can be done on all parts of the body. In my case, it was done through my Crown Chakra, which is located at the top of the head.

The biggest challenge in working through the Crown Chakra is mental, especially when someone is too withdrawn, attached to the materialistic pursuits of existence, or stuck in their way of thinking. A person with a blocked Crown Chakra may be unwilling to open themselves to other ideas, thoughts, or knowledge. When the Crown Chakra is unbalanced, a person can experience psychosis, dissociation, and a general feeling of being disconnected or ungrounded.

Levon would simply place his hands above my Crown Chakra and slowly draw energy out of my body and into his before releasing it into a bowl of salt water. During this healing process, my head moved back and forth, which Levon said was inevitable.

Throughout, I had to think positively, as that plays a big role in the process. The burning incense and soft meditation music relaxed me, which helped my mind let go. I noticed that when I was tense, the incense smoke rose in curls, but once I was relaxed, the smoke rose upward gently and smoothly. Reiki can become a part of your mind and soul, but only if you allow it to. There is positive and negative energy. To grasp the positive energy, you must believe in

Reiki and be convinced of its effectiveness. When I started taking my herbs, I quickly came to believe in Reiki and all it entails. It came to exist within me. More importantly, I started to believe in myself. This was another piece of hope I could hold on to.

I also tried acupuncture to help with my seizures. According to the Pacific College of Health and Science, an institute of higher learning that specializes in alternative medicine, Chinese acupuncture helps restore the flow of *qi*, or energy, throughout the body. *Qi* flows along pathways known as meridians and plays an important role in the body's functioning. In a person without epilepsy, the flow of *qi* is—or should be—balanced. In an individual with epilepsy, the flow of *qi* is believed to be impeded. Traditional Chinese Medicine (TCM) and acupuncture aim to restore the unimpeded flow of *qi* throughout the body. To restore the flow of *qi*, an acupuncturist inserts tiny needles into certain points in the body, which allows them to access the meridians through which *qi* flows.

The lady who performed acupuncture for me placed tiny needles in the center of my head, the center of my forehead, the crack above my lip, the center of my elbow, and in my stomach. The needles in my head, forehead, and lip were a bit uncomfortable when first inserted.

In an individual with epilepsy, the acupuncturist then manipulates key points within the body believed to increase the flow of *qi* to the head. Once the flow of *qi* has been restored, it is essential that it is maintained in its balanced state. An acupuncturist may recommend certain herbs and dietary products to help keep the *qi* in its natural state. I followed the recommended diet for a few months, but it didn't seem to have any effect for me.

I never considered traditional 'talk' therapy, but Lara, in Jerusalem, encouraged me to try energy healing through attunement therapy. This is how I met Jeffrey Goldstein (Jeff), a remarkable attunement instructor and therapist who offers spiritual guidance and is also a somatic experience practitioner. He helped me a great deal, and I learned a lot from him. He believes in peace and conducts workshops on his healing practices and emotional wellness aids with organizations in Palestine.

Attunement is the spiritual practice of opening one's thoughts and feelings to the source of wisdom and love. It is a healing modality offered through the hands, though without touch. This is how Jeff describes attunement:

> *Attunement is a method of Energy Therapy that helps to bring the body into homeostasis by nurturing, relaxing, and therefore regulating the body's systems. It also helps the nervous system to restart or renew itself into the present moment and it affects the electromagnetic patterns within the brain waves.*
>
> *This is excellent for those afflicted with epilepsy, because of the vast dysregulation that is created in the nervous system.*
>
> *Janine took advantage of this state of relaxation, which assisted her to feel better about herself when she had an attack.*

At the time, only two people knew I was going to attunement therapy: Lara, who joined me for my first session, and Allison, who took me a few times after that. I didn't want anyone else to know that I was even trying this, and I'm not really sure why. I just kept it to myself. Now, I can't say enough about how important it was—and still is—to me. I often recommend it to people in the hope that they will benefit and get as much from it as I do. Even after becoming seizure free, I still go to attunement therapy, and with my seizures gone, I am more relaxed and benefit a lot from it.

The brain is a complex organ. It is constantly at work, sending electrical signals, communicating, building new neural connections, and so on. This electrical activity, also known as brainwaves, reflects our state of mind. Our reality is not based on outside influences; it is an internal process based on our thoughts, perceptions, and emotions. If we can deepen our understanding of these brainwaves, we can control our reality.

Our brainwaves have five frequencies: beta, alpha, theta, delta, and gamma. It is entirely natural for humans to experience these different states at different times of the day, though one state is generally dominant.

The theta brainwave frequency is the one in which the body and mind's natural self-healing processes are activated and optimized. Theta brainwaves are present during deep relaxation, dreaming, meditation, and hypnosis. They can be a source of creativity, intuition, increased memory, and enhanced concentration. When these brain waves are induced through certain mental practices, they lower stress and anxiety levels and facilitate healing and growth. Accessing the theta frequency of brainwaves allows us to act below the level of the conscious mind, in the first stage of the dream state. This facilitates the ideal mental and physiological state for healing, and it also enables us to access the power and wisdom of our unconscious mind, which is normally inaccessible in more alert states.

Receiving attunement meant I was healing myself from within. It is the most profound healing therapy I've ever experienced. We all have the ability to heal ourselves, but attunement therapy helps awaken the soul. We are all made up of energy, and it flows through us. We don't actually see it, but it's there. It is the energy of our life force. This energy comes from the Universal Source—the highest power in your belief system—and is channeled by the attunement practitioner, flowing through them to the receiver.

Attunement is more sensing, less thinking, and I found this type of therapy to be very powerful. It helped me find peace with myself and with my disorder so my thoughts and feelings could stop fighting each other. It enabled me to break free of the endless negative, even suicidal, thoughts that plagued me. I found the healing sessions to be extremely relaxing and very therapeutic.

I would go into a deep state of stillness, where emotions could be released. Then, my subconscious mind carried me to the places that needed healing. In stillness, I would reach inward and listen to the voice hidden inside me. All I had to do was close my eyes and relax. Almost immediately, I would feel a warmth and a tingling sensation of gentle energy flow. This experience differs from one person to another. Some feel a deep, calm relaxation, others have a whole host of different experiences and sensations, as I did. I believed in the process, and therefore, it had a strong positive effect on me.

I gave myself permission to open and release all the trapped energy that had been locked up inside my body and help it melt away. On many occasions, I felt like my body was completely surrounded by a protective bubble of light. Attunement made me feel like I was free. I regard it as a form of spiritual guidance. I didn't want to let it overtake me, and it wasn't a replacement for my Christianity, which I believe in strongly, but it helped me a great deal.

During my second attunement healing session, while wrapped in a deep stillness, I noticed my legs very slowly tucking in toward my stomach, as if I were a fetus in a womb. I assumed this was because I was seeking help for my epilepsy, which began when I was a baby. When I told Allison—who was in the room the whole time—about this experience and the suspected causes behind it, she said, "Your body didn't move. You were lying still throughout the whole attunement session and there were tears."

I later learned that experience was part of what is known as Theta Healing. In Theta Healing, you imagine yourself floating up above your head through your Crown Chakra to ask God for help. When this happens, your brainwaves instantly shift into the theta range, the realm of the subconscious. This holds our memories, including our memories of sensations. It also governs our attitudes, beliefs, and behaviors.

Lorine joined me once to see what an attunement therapy session looked like. She didn't know what to expect, since she didn't entirely believe what I told her about my previous experiences. What she saw amazed her so much that it took her a few days to make sense of it all.

During that session, I released a lot of anger. I clenched my fists, and tears rolled down my cheeks endlessly. Lorine was able to see these reactions because my motor neurons kicked in. Motor neurons are found in the nervous system and activate muscle cells. They carry information from the central nervous system to the muscle cells, telling my fists to clench. This happened while I was in deep meditative state. My mind and body were communicating with each other. I would open my arms wide and feel at peace. Then, suddenly, I would feel my fists start to clench in anger. Then, the process would repeat; I'd reopen my arms in very slow motion, and a feeling of peace would return. I was releasing all the anguish and rage that had formed deep inside me.

Attunement sessions aren't all like that. Sometimes, the body can feel something happening, but it doesn't necessarily move, which is what happened with Allison during my second experience with attunement.

During theta brainwave activity, both the body and mind experience enhanced rejuvenation, growth, and healing. Due to the deep levels of relaxation that theta brainwaves facilitate, the body and mind can more easily restore themselves during and after illness, as well as after mental burnout and physical exertion.

With attunement, I found an easier way to release my pent-up body emotions. The body never forgets, and my subconscious was full of sustained, long-term pain and intense mental suffering, both from the fact of having seizures and also from the side effects of my medications to control the seizures.

After the session she observed, Lorine said to me, "All these years I've known you, I never knew how much pain you've hidden and felt inside. All I've ever seen in you is strength and like Jeff said, you don't see your strength."

A few years after my surgery, I was reflecting on my journey one day and began to cry. I needed to thank everyone who had helped me over the years, and I ended up sending them a very emotional voice message. Later, when Lorine brought it up, I realized that I had probably made her cry with my outpouring of emotions, though she doesn't cry easily. To lighten the mood, I followed up with, "Ha ha, I bet that made you cry."

She replied, "That didn't make me cry. The only time I cried for you was when I saw your reactions during your attunement session, when you released all that pain you've been holding inside, which you hid so well."

That's why this incident made her cry when nothing else having to do with me ever had. She felt such sympathy for what I was going through on the inside. She couldn't believe what was happening before her very eyes. She saw how real it was and that I wasn't putting on an act.

I felt the same way during my first few attunement sessions; I couldn't believe what was happening while it was happening to me. I could feel what was happening, but I wasn't the one doing it. That's why I decided to learn everything there is to know about attunement—because of its realness. I wanted to justify what I was experiencing, why it was happening, and why others were able to witness what I was experiencing.

Attunement helped me relax and release, but it didn't control my seizures. It may work that way for some people, but for me, it was more about emotional and psychological wellness.

I continued working with Jeff, and in time, I was able to release all my emotional bodily memories. He made a big difference in my life and freed me from so much past pain. After I completed my healing journey, I created a token of appreciation for him so he would know just how much he helped me. It speaks to how powerful attunement therapy was for me:

to see if I got any seizures since I would then only be taking one medication, Lamictal.

I waited impatiently for the six months to pass, and when they finally did, I didn't hear anything more about my license. I kept telling myself, "I'll receive the call any day now, or something will surely arrive in the mail." But nothing did. I tried calling them countless times until I finally got through to an operator, whom I hoped would speak English or Arabic. They didn't. I wasn't about to hang up, though, because I had been on hold for almost half an hour, so I ran downstairs to see if my neighbor Hania's daughter, Khuloud, was home because I knew she spoke Hebrew. Thankfully, she was there. She spoke to them on my behalf, and the lady told her that they had sent me something by registered mail at the end of July—which was the six-month mark—but she couldn't tell me what it was and insisted I had to go to the office in person, since I never received the document. It was now September of 2017, and it doesn't take two months for internal registered mail to arrive, so it must've gotten lost.

The problem was that their office was in Tel Aviv, forty-five minutes away, and I couldn't just pick up and go anytime I wanted. I didn't have an appointment, and Dimitri worked during their office hours. I was frustrated and had been waiting impatiently, so I asked Dimitri to take a day off to take me there. I would take my chances with not having an appointment.

A few days later, Dimitri took the day off, and we went to the Road and Safety Department in Tel Aviv. I knocked on the guard's window, and he simply wouldn't allow me to set foot inside without an appointment. I gave him my ID to give to the receptionist and tried to communicate the missing mail situation, but he could only speak Hebrew. I was insistent, though, and kept trying to communicate with him. I didn't know that he had access to the computers and was practically begging him to find a way to help me get inside. In the end, I guess he decided to give me a break and just entered my information into the computer to see if that would help him understand what I wanted. Luckily, he saw the information that had been sent in the mail—information that could've easily been communicated over the phone. Since we couldn't communicate properly, he reached out for my mobile phone. I didn't understand what he was doing at first, but using the Hebrew keyboard, he wrote down what was written in my file: "Go to the driver's license office." I knew then that I was getting my license back. I wanted to hug him.

If I had never driven before and didn't know the feeling of independence and freedom that comes with it, I wouldn't have felt so strongly about driving or been so eager to get my license back. Some people don't drive by choice, and that is fine. But even the people who tried to convince me that not being able to drive wasn't a big deal admitted they couldn't imagine themselves going seven and a half years without driving!

When I finally went to get my license back, the same lady who had taken it away gave it back to me. Despite her unassuming appearance, I could pick her out of a police line-up. I'll never be able to forget her face when I first surrendered my license to her. My license still had a year left before it expired, which was great. I drove back home, and Dimitri was thrilled to be sitting in the passenger seat because he hates driving. Of course, I'm sure he was sitting on the edge of his seat, considering I hadn't driven in so long. The next day, I was already running errands. From then on, I was the one behind the wheel almost every day, and I drove during all our family outings.

Chapter Twenty-Five

I have always loved to write, so I poured my heartache onto paper by writing poetry. I wrote my first poem in university. I called it "Only If" and wrote it for Nadine, though I never shared it with her. The first time she read it was in this book.

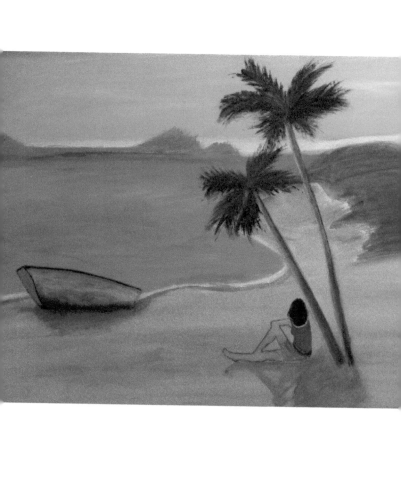

Only If

The sky is clear, the night is young
there's no one in sight, merely the moon looking down
Alone I stand along the ocean side, my heart overthrown
on sand
surpassing me a soft cool breeze, a beautiful scene it was
to see

Only if there could've been another one present

Towards the ocean I must go, to see where my future is
leading me
trying to release my deep-seated thoughts into the open
fresh air
I find myself sitting on the moist sand with my arms
wrapped around my legs
looking out towards the empty peaceful view

Only if there could've been another one present

The seat of passion within me is exhaled in a raging
outburst
as I take a long deep breath, all the agony disappears
That same breath quietens all the anguish inside
there I remain alone yet again, only this time with a feeling
of relief

Only if there could've been another one present

Left alone, I never am
She was always the one present.

throughout the whole family, with everyone asking if anyone had heard from me. I once joked about this to Allison, who probably didn't believe me. But then, one time, she had my mobile sitting next to her during my attunement session, and when I was done, she said, "Oh my God, the whole world really did send you messages and call you!" I wasn't kidding. My family's love, patience, and tolerance was my greatest support during my battle with epilepsy. It made me feel accepted, gave me a ray of hope, and most importantly, gave me a reason to live and to continue fighting.

When I finally became seizure free, I realized that my hobbies of photography, painting, writing poetry, putting together puzzles, walking, playing squash, kickboxing, and swimming was my own form of therapy. They kept me going and helped me stay sane and positive.

One time, Soula and I were at Marwa's house having a coffee in Jericho. Nibal, a girl whom I vaguely knew through Tarek and Samer, came over as well. We had bumped into each other on many occasions, and her son Andre had been one of Joseph's classmates and friend for years, but we didn't know much about each others' personal lives. We were all chatting over coffee when Nibal said, "I saw your painting on Facebook. I didn't know you liked to paint."

I said, "Yes, I've been painting for years."

Soula turned to me and said with a chuckle, "Janine, be careful! She's trying to analyze you."

I smiled. "That's fine. She can do all the analyzing she wants." The painting I had posted was of a simple abstract design, not one you can really read much into.

At some point during our conversation, I remembered that Nibal had once mentioned that she was studying art therapy. That's when I understood what Soula meant with her comment about Nibal "analyzing" me. However, she wasn't and had no intention of doing so.

Being the social butterfly that I am, I started to make conversation with her, which eventually led to asking her about the whole art therapy course she was doing. I knew what art therapy was, but having a passion for art, I was interested in hearing exactly what she was doing. She started telling me about her coursework and what she still needed to do to get her degree. She said, "I'm about to start working on a case study research paper that explores how different things can be expressed through art, how you can read a person's emotions or struggles through art, and so on."

At this point, Nibal had no idea that most of my paintings were part of my own art therapy while I was still having seizures. I saw an opportunity to help her. I said, "Would you like to do your research paper on art therapy and epilepsy? I wouldn't mind being your case study."

At that moment, she didn't know that she had just hit the jackpot, but I knew. I knew my paintings were exactly what she was looking for. All I cared about was helping her, since it was for a good cause.

When she later called to interview me, I answered all her questions. Then, she asked me to send her some of my paintings, and I did. Actually, that's all I did; she did everything else on her own. I was merely a subject for her to work with. I was so happy for her when she told me that she passed with the highest grade in the class.

Nibal recalls her work with me:

had already asked Dr. Imad if we could discuss my seizures with him.

I was always researching new treatments for seizures in hopes of avoiding brain surgery, and I had recently discovered the Vagus Nerve Stimulation (VNS) device. It's like a pacemaker, but for the brain. The VNS device is surgically implanted under the skin in the upper left part of the chest. An electrode or wire is attached to the device, and the wire is wound around the vagus nerve in the neck. It prevents or decreases the number of seizures by stimulating the vagus nerve with electrical impulses. People with VNS devices don't even notice them working. If a person does feel a seizure coming on, they can swipe a magnet over the device to send an additional burst of stimulation to the brain, which might help stop the seizure. It comes with many side effects immediately after surgery, like difficulty swallowing, voice change, shortness of breath, and more, but for me, they sounded bearable, especially when compared to brain surgery.

I was so convinced that this would work for me and that it would be the perfect solution. However, when I brought up the VNS device to Dr. Imad, he said it wasn't an acceptable option for complex-partial seizures. It felt like a punch in the gut.

Once again, I was left with no other option except brain surgery, which he discussed with me in detail. He assured me that it was a very good option and had successful results. He then graciously emailed me a list of neurosurgeons around the world whom he knew and recommended performing surgery. He also said I could use his name as reference. King Faisal Specialty Hospital is only for Saudi patients; otherwise, with his qualifications and vast experience in his field, I wouldn't think twice about having him perform my brain surgery. However, surgery for me was out of the question. I was too afraid that it wouldn't work and that I'd be left blind, with memory loss, and dealing with a host of other horrible side effects.

Years later, when I finally did decide to proceed with the surgery, it was important to me that I tell him of my decision. I wanted him to know that I was following his advice, even though I hadn't back then. So, I sent him an email telling him about it, and his reply was as generous as ever. He asked me to send him my test results by express mail so he could review them and stay on top of the case. He always readily advised me on how to proceed with my treatment and played a major and very important role in my journey. I deeply appreciate it and will forever treasure him.

In 2012, during my follow-up appointment with Dr. Dana, she gave me the same advice Dr. Imad had the year before: she told me that I should consider the surgery option, since my seizures weren't being controlled by medication and were only getting worse. I wasn't ready for this advice when it first came up, nor was I ready for it now. Once again, I refused.

Dimitri had already read everything he could about the surgery and was very much in favor of it, but the decision, he said, was totally mine. There were pros and cons to the surgery, but only I could weigh them; no one could make that decision for me. I always came back to him with questions: "What about you and the boys? How could I take a risk like this? I might end up getting brain damage, and you three would then have to take care of me for the rest of my life! I would never want that for any of you. What if I lose my memory? I couldn't bear the thought of not being able to recognize you and the boys. What you're all going through is already enough. I don't want to be a burden on you all for the rest of your lives."

Dr. Imad and Dr. Dana were both giving me the best medical advice. I just wasn't ready to take the risk of brain surgery.

My parents didn't give up hope of finding another option. They continued to take me to all kinds of different doctors in hopes of finding another solution. They even took me to Geneva to visit a professor there who was recommended by another friend, but he had no other solutions except to wait for a new medication to come out on the market and see if that could control my seizures.

Another cousin, Faten, knew a senior neurologist, Dr. Steve, who was based in Dubai. She said to me, "While you're visiting your parents, why don't you go see him?" She kindly got in touch with him and scheduled an appointment for me to see him during my stay in Dubai.

He walked into our meeting and said, "Okay, I don't need to ask you any questions. Just tell me your story from A-Z."

I started from day one and told him my entire history of epilepsy, the different medications I'd tried, and different specialists I'd seen.

When I was done, he said, "So, when you were living in Miami, Dr. Patrick told you that you're a great candidate for surgery. How long ago was that?" Before I could even answer, he continued, "That was 1998! It's now 2014, and you've tried five different medications, all without success. Your seizures are clearly drug-resistant and only going to get worse with time. What are you waiting for? Don't you think it's time?"

His words gave me the final push I needed. That night, I told Dimitri that I was going to see Dr. Dana when we got back to Jerusalem, and that's exactly what I did.

I explained to her that when she first recommended surgery, I didn't give it any serious thought because I was worried about being a burden on Dimitri and my boys. She said, "It's actually quite the opposite. You shouldn't worry about them if you have the surgery, but you should worry about them if you don't." She pointed out that my seizures were already getting worse and explained that they could spread into the center of my brain. If that happened, surgery would no longer be an option. That's when Dimitri and the boys would end up taking care of me. My age was another reason not to wait because the procedure becomes more dangerous as you get older. At that point, I was thirty-seven years old. Since my seizures started when I was thirteen, I had been suffering from them for twenty-four years.

She set up an appointment for me a few days later to meet with her and the neurosurgeon, Professor Moni Benifla, Head of the Pediatric Neurosurgery Unit and Epilepsy Surgeon. He has spent his career teaching and specializing in pediatric brain tumors, epilepsy, congenital malformations of the central nervous system, and head trauma.

He discussed the procedure with me and detailed the relatively impressive success rates. Then, he said, "I hate to say this, but there is a 1 percent death rate." I froze. Before I could respond, he added, "You could get run over by a car tomorrow, too." That was a good point.

I suddenly recalled an accident I was in years earlier with Nadine, Nisreen, and Nada, which almost cost us our lives. We planned a getaway trip to Lebanon, where Nada was living at the time.

One evening during our trip, Nada picked us up, and we all went out and enjoyed a girl's night out in Beirut. On our way back to the hotel, a girl ran a stop sign and crashed into us in the intersection. Nada's car spun at least five times at a very high speed before hitting a jeep parked next to the sidewalk. That's what finally got our car to stop spinning.

Once the car came to a complete stop, there was a moment of silence. Then, there was a harsh, strident sound, and the back window dropped down and shattered due to the powerful crash. Pieces of glass scattered all over the back seat. I remember noticing the jeep's forest-green color.

The four of us were silent and sat frozen in place, as if life had been put on pause. I had my head tucked between my legs and my hands above my head. I'll never forget my reaction at that moment. I lifted my head slowly and asked if anyone was dead. We were all in shock. Everyone in the streets rushed over and helped us out of the car. There was a small hotel nearby, so one guy went in and got us some water and ice.

After we collected ourselves, we looked over to see what happened to the other driver. The girl who ran the stop sign was fine. In fact, she was ranting and raving about how angry her father was going to be because she'd banged up her Porsche. That's all she cared about.

It was definitely one of the scarier moments of my life. But was it really comparable to brain surgery?

I listened to everything Dr. Moni had to say, then went home and did my own research as well. After all, it was my brain they'd be digging into.

The most common and best-understood procedure for my type of seizures is referred to as a 'resection of tissue in the temporal lobe.' Although, the results vary, as many as 70 percent of people who undergo this procedure no longer experience seizures that make them lose consciousness or have convulsions. A few do still experience an aura, but they don't have the seizure itself. Up to 20 percent of patients still experience some seizures but find that their symptoms and frequency are greatly reduced; this group has an approximately 85 percent reduction in seizures. Between 10 and 15 percent of patients show little-to-no improvement. All said, about 85 percent of people who undergo this type of surgery see improvement in their seizures. According to Dr. Dana, on average, their facility did twenty-to-twenty-five of these surgeries each year.

Between 2014-2015, I did all the tests required before surgery. Altogether, it was about eight tests.

Normally, you can't get an MRI overnight. Luckily, I could, because my dad is very good friends with a well-known and respected doctor in Jerusalem, Dr. Basem Abuasab, who is also the CEO of Alhayat Medical Centers in Jerusalem. He got me in for an appointment much, much sooner than the general public could. This was critical, because I knew that if I had too much time to think about the surgery, I might back out.

But that didn't happen. I felt ready. It was my time. God gave me strength. I am very grateful to Dr. Basem for all his help and continuous support to this day.

When I finally left the hospital, Dimitri's sister, Dima, helped me remove the glue from my hair. She was so patient with me, because the glue was pasted onto my scalp, and after being glued on for so long, it was practically stuck. It took her almost two hours because she was being very careful not to hurt me or pluck out my hair.

Functional MRI

A functional MRI is a noninvasive technique for measuring and mapping brain activity. It is used to understand how the normal function of the brain is disrupted by disease.

With this test, I had to go into the MRI machine with my head secured inside a hard plastic mask which was placed around my head and it covered my face from above. It was very uncomfortable, and it made me feel claustrophobic. I also had to wear a pair of thick goggles similar to the ones used for virtual reality. These displayed instructions for me digitally. I was given a button to hold in my left hand and instructed to press it while answering questions silently. Unfortunately, English wasn't an option, so the questions were being asked in classic Arabic, and there was a lot of information in this test. I also had to lie completely still, which was a bit nerve-racking. I couldn't wait for the lady behind the microphone to say it was over.

Neuropsychological Evaluation

A neuropsychological evaluation is a test to measure how well a person's brain is working. The abilities tested include reading, language usage, attention, learning, processing speed, reasoning, memory, problem-solving, mood, personality, and more.

For this test, a psychologist came and talked with me.

He asked me to tell him about myself. Then, he had me go on to another topic. After a few minutes, he suddenly stopped me and asked me about something I'd said ten minutes prior. It was a constant back and forth, and every time I started to figure out the conversation's pattern, he surprised me with something new.

This was intended to make sure my memory and concentration were working formally. He also wanted to check whether I was mentally ready for the surgery. Little did he know, I was readier than ever.

a joke about it. I was fearless and very calm. Later that day, a different nurse came and asked me a few questions, such as whether I smoked or drank heavily. These kinds of things would affect my anesthesia dosage prior to the surgery.

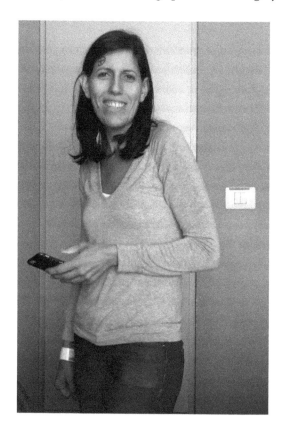

The day of the surgery, they woke me up at 5 a.m. to do an electrocardiogram (EKG) to check for signs of heart disease.

The surgery was scheduled for 7 a.m. When I reached the operating room, an intern brought me some papers to sign. He explained that they were for me to legally agree to the surgery and all the risks that came with it. Looking down at the black line where I was told to sign, two thoughts crossed my mind. First, "Am I signing my own death certificate?" And second, "It's now or never!" At that point, it was a leap of faith.

I signed.

immediately agreed, he quipped, "Where would you like me to send it?" I said, "Somewhere where there's sunshine and beaches." He chuckled and said, "I'll see what I can do."

After a pause, I added, "Make sure you don't cut the wrong vein." I couldn't help but imagine a scene in an action movie where the hero is disarming a bomb and isn't sure whether to cut the red or blue wire.

They wheeled me into the preparation room. It was a very small room, just wide enough to fit the bed and two other people. The walls were covered in cabinets and compartments, and as the nurses bustled around me, I saw that these were full of needles, swabs, gloves, and equipment—everything needed for surgery. One of the nurses started injecting me with various needles and inserted a catheter. Then, I saw the razor behind her. I already knew they were going to have to shave my head, but I was still worried about it. When she was done, she said, "Don't worry. I didn't take away too much of your hair."

I'd wanted to get a haircut before the surgery, but Dimitri suggested I wait until afterward so I could see what I still had to work with. Luckily, the nurse told the truth: she took very little hair. She shaved a huge question mark design into my head, which looked odd at first. Eventually, my hair grew back, and the question mark became hidden. The only way to see it now is to search through my hair for the scar. It's funny: at the time, I was so worried about losing a chunk of my hair, and now, I wouldn't mind walking around bald and showing it off. That scar represents the best decision I ever made. It reminds me of how brave I was.

I was now ready to enter the operating room. This was a huge room, and there were about four people inside, other than Dr. Moni, all preparing for the surgery. One of them was the intern who brought me the final paperwork. He had already told me that he was looking forward to being part of the team inside the OR. He was so happy about it and went on about how everything would be okay. There was also a second neurology intern whom I hadn't met before who was going to be present for the surgery. I didn't worry too much about that. After all, how else could they become surgeons without observing and assisting with the real thing?

All too soon, I was staring up at the high white ceiling and the bright lights surrounding me. I began silently praying that I would make it out of the surgery alive and not have any complications during or after the surgery. The anesthesiologist was getting ready to put me to sleep. I was starting to get nervous, but he was cheerful and whistling in a hushed tone, trying to make the atmosphere less scary and more relaxed. He told me to think of somewhere green, like a beautiful meadow, and imagine myself there. He had me start counting down from ten. By eight, the bright lights were starting to dim. By six, I was out like a light.

Right before the anesthesia shot, I had a seizure. The clock on the wall showed that it was 8:13 a.m. It was the last seizure I ever had. My twenty-five-year journey with epilepsy ended at the age of thirty-eight on October 29, 2015.

The surgery I had was called an amygdalohippocampectomy. In the past, the surgical treatment for temporal lobe epilepsy—the most common form of epileptic seizures that originate from a single point in the brain—involved removing the entire anterior portion of the temporal lobe, called an anterior temporal lobectomy. The more selective amygdalohippocampectomy spares the unaffected portion of the anterior temporal lobe.

In a selective amygdalohippocampectomy, the following portions of the medial temporal lobe are removed:

237

just minutes after they first rolled me into the ICU. I wasn't allowed to have visitors yet, so he snuck in with someone else going to see another patient but got caught and had to leave.

Little by little, Uncle Yousef; Aunt Antoinette; Aunt Janet; Edgar; Dima; my aunts Anisa and Salwa; and my uncles Maurice and Samir all started coming in a few at a time.

While I was still in the ICU, I underwent a CT scan because there was a little bleeding in my brain. There was also some air between the incision and the brain. Of course, Dimitri wasted no time in calling me an airhead! As Dr. Dana explained, this was perfectly normal after the type of surgery I'd undergone, but the hospital staff still had to keep a close eye on it.

This is what the Epilepsy Foundation has to say about brain surgery recovery:

> In general, recovery after epilepsy surgery can take weeks to months. Though the hospital stay may be only a few days, it takes longer for the brain to heal, especially if an open surgery was done. In the first week after surgery, people may have headaches, have an upset stomach, and feel tired. There may be temporary swelling of the forehead and area around the eye, as well as jaw pain on the side of surgery. People are usually given medication after surgery to help limit these post-surgical symptoms.
>
> Most people are back to school or work in 4 to 6 weeks. Gradually easing back into normal activities is best. It may take several months for a person's attention span, thinking, or memory to reach baseline after surgery.

The morphine started wearing off the night of the surgery, and I was in a lot of pain, so the nurse gave me more morphine in the middle of the night, which helped me sleep. Then, the next morning, she gave me regular painkillers because she couldn't give me any more morphine. That's when the real pain struck, but it was worth it. I knew the pain would soon be forgotten. I don't know why, but the morning after my surgery, my intuition told me that I was finally free of my seizures. I just knew it was over.

That same morning, Dima wrote a heartfelt Facebook post about my surgery. She praised God, added a snapshot of me smiling that was taken a few months before the surgery, and tagged me in the post. A few people misinterpreted it for an Arab obituary. Some people were giving their condolences in the comments, others were asking how I'd died, and a few were confused because they had just heard of my surgery's success. My parents' phones wouldn't stop ringing. Dima quickly edited her post to put everyone's minds at ease.

The first few days after the surgery were tough, but I was slowly healing. The swelling around my eyes gradually went down, and the bruising colors started to change. I didn't have much of an appetite, but I sometimes ate a bit of soup.

I was in the ICU for five days, then a regular room for two days. Once again, my mom didn't leave my side and slept over the entire time I was in the hospital and she and my dad stayed in Jerusalem throughout my recovery period.

Nadine could only stay for a week after my surgery because she had left Eddie, Natalie, and Carl in Qatar. As she was heading home, I called her to tell her that I was being discharged from the hospital.

I stayed at my parents' house for the first two weeks of recovery while Dimitri and the boys slept at home. He came over after work each day, and the boys came over after

Johnny recalls my surgery as being a difficult time for him:

When my mom had the surgery, I slept on her pillow every night until she came home. She would always remind me of how she would be okay, but I was in pain every day. I try not to remember all this. But I remember going in that hospital room with needles and machines all around her and my mom just smiling and it was the best thing that happened. I would leave anybody and anything to go visit her. If my dad said we're going to see mom, I'd be ready in two seconds.

I'm sure my appearance was terrifying and didn't help the boys feel better. My incision was stitched together with a very thick thread that was akin to a plastic wire. The skin of the scalp is very sensitive, and the wire ensured that the wound would stay closed.

Sometimes when I talked a lot, my lower lip would slightly droop on the right side, causing my speech to become a bit heavy and slurred. This was caused by the tight wire stitches pulling the skin on the right side of my face. It was best not to talk a lot, but being the chatterbox that I am, that was incredibly difficult for me.

The first time this happened was in the hospital the day after my surgery. Everyone in the room froze; they thought I was having a seizure. Before I could assure Nadine that it wasn't a seizure, she had already rushed out to get the nurse.

After the surgery, the upper right side of my face above my cheekbone was a tiny bit higher than my left side, but the swelling went down within a few months. Only an inward curve on the right side of my forehead remains. I only know it's there because it wasn't present before surgery; otherwise, it's barely noticeable. The scar line at the end of the incision beside my right ear has also faded. Still, these small elements of my appearance didn't matter to me then and don't matter to me now. All that matters is that I am seizure free.

I returned to the hospital a week after I was discharged to have them remove the stitches. It was absolute hell getting them out. The area was both very sensitive and completely numb.

I also asked Dr. Moni if I had a metal plate in my head that would set off alarms while going through security at the airport. He said, "No, it's made of titanium, which won't set off alarms. You're very expensive."

I have a certificate affirming my condition for when I go through the airport, but I've never set off an alarm, so I haven't needed to show it.

If you aren't comfortable looking at photos of surgery or the post-surgical results, please skip the next page.

With the success of my surgery, Rinal decided to go forward with it as well. She had to go through all the tests, which takes a long time. It can take months just to get an appointment for an MRI! My six-month follow-up MRI was coming up, so I tried to give her my appointment. I knew it might not work, but it wouldn't hurt to try. I didn't want Rinal to backpedal during the long testing process. I know what it's like to be terrified and start doubting your decision.

I called the hospital's appointment center and asked if they could switch my appointment to hers. The lady I spoke with said they could only cancel, not switch, my appointment. After half an hour of arguing and being put on hold, she was finally convinced that it was for an important cause and that I wasn't asking much. The only problem was that she didn't have the authority to make this change. I said, "Fine, I understand, but please let me speak to the person who does have the authority. Otherwise, you'll end up losing two patients. I won't cancel it, no one will show up, and the appointment will go to waste." She transferred me to someone who could make the requested change. After another fifteen minutes of arguing with him, he agreed to replace my ID number with hers in the appointment. I was so happy; now, Rinal's surgery could be done much earlier than planned.

Rinal's surgery took place a year after mine, and she remains seizure free to this day.

A year after my surgery, Dr. Dana asked me if she could give my mobile number to one of her patients who was considering having the same surgery. It took this lady more than two months to call me. She didn't give me her name, and I didn't ask. She didn't want me to know who she was. She simply said, "You were referred to me by Dr. Dana." We spoke for at least an hour. I gave her the best advice I could but was careful not to give her false hope. I detailed the advantages of the surgery, its success rates, and the many ways it changed my life for the better. I assured her that it was worth the risk and that it was the best decision I ever made. She told me that her seizures only happened at night while she was asleep, so she had many sleepless nights and was often exhausted the next day at work. She wanted me to make the decision for her, since I had done it already. Again and again, she asked me if I thought she should have the surgery and if it would work. I kept telling her that it was a decision only she could make; no one else could make it for her.

For a few seconds, I thought, "Lucky her! She only has seizures at night. She can lead a normal life during the day. She can drive. No one would even know she has seizures." But that was foolish and unfair of me; I had no idea what her life was really like. Much of my reaction was based on the fact that she could still drive, an activity that meant so much to me.

I wrongly assumed that she was better off having her seizures at night, rather than during the day. I hated myself for even thinking that, however briefly. I know that lack of sleep is one of the most common triggers for seizures, so even though she didn't have seizures during the day, it didn't mean her life was easier than mine. She may well have woken up each morning lying in a puddle of her own urine. She could get seriously injured by falling out of bed. What's worse, she could choke on her own saliva during the seizure if she were lying flat on her back.

I've had a few seizures during my sleep, and it really is a horrible experience. After I woke up, I was gasping for breath and very confused. When Nadine and I moved to Miami from North Carolina during university, we didn't live in the dorms anymore. My dad bought us a two-

reduced the brightness of my screen, sat a little further back, and took occasional breaks from the screen to give my eyes a rest. These days, you can use a monitor glare guard, wear non-glare glasses, or buy a flicker-free monitor.

I did everything I could to prevent a seizure from happening by monitoring myself and being aware of my triggers, but many of my seizures happened for no clear reason. I didn't want my seizures to get in my way of doing what I wanted, but since they were uncontrolled, I had to make compromises at times.

My epilepsy journey didn't end with my surgery. If anything, I became an important part of many other peoples' epilepsy journeys.

This began when Fatima sent me a message about her colleague in Saudi Arabia whose twelve-year-old daughter suffered from epilepsy. Fatima had told her colleague about my surgery, and she wanted to learn more. She hadn't even known there was a surgery that could treat seizures. I agreed to talk to her about my experience. Once again, I didn't set out to convince her, but I told her everything she needed to know to make her own decision.

The first thing I told her was that this surgery was not for everyone and that the required tests would confirm whether or not her daughter was a candidate for the proce-dure. I explained the reasons for this to the best of my ability and knowledge.

She then asked if I knew of any other hospitals abroad that could perform this procedure. There are entry restric-tions in Israel, and she and her daughter would have a very hard time just getting into the country. I recommended Cleveland Clinic in Ohio in the US, as Dr. Imad had previ-ously recommended it to me. Cleveland Clinic's Neurology and Neurosurgery program is one of the top-ranked programs in the US. I told her that her daughter would have to go through a thorough medical and physical examination at their clinic, not in Saudi Arabia, so they could decide whether she was a candidate for surgery. I then explained the surgical procedure itself, the recovery period, and its outcome.

We stayed in touch for a while, and then, I stopped hearing from her. I didn't follow up because I didn't want to impose myself. Still, I was curious about what she and her daughter decided and whether the daughter was a candidate for surgery. About a year later, I asked Fatima if she knew anything about it, but she had lost touch with the mother, too.

In February of 2018, Dr. Dana asked me if she could give my number to an association that was looking for someone who spoke both English and Arabic. I said yes, I wouldn't mind at all.

A few days later, a gentleman called me from the Eyal Epilepsy Association and told me that they needed someone who could write content for their website in both English and Arabic from scratch. I agreed and asked Dimitri if he could help me translate my writing from English to Arabic. There was no official deadline, but I gave myself my own deadline. I worked while the boys were at school, so I wouldn't be taking time away from them when they got home. It took a little over a month, but I met my self-imposed deadline. However, I couldn't rush Dimitri since he was doing the translation work as a favor for me when he had a little free time. Instead, the association suggested they hire an Arabic translator.

I already knew a great deal about the topics I was covering, yet I still learned some new things along the way. I found that I enjoyed the work.

done with them, he gave them to me for future use. He even offered to provide a meeting hall and hot and cold refreshments for a public event I was planning in November for Epilepsy Awareness Month.

During a follow-up visit with Dr. Dana, I gave her some of the flyers to give to her patients and asked her if it would be possible for her to send out a group message to all her patients inviting them to attend the event I was planning. She said, "This is such an amazing thing you're doing, but we're no longer allowed to do that. We'd be slapped with a lawsuit. You know what's sad, though? Even if I was allowed to send out messages, most people wouldn't come because they wouldn't want to reveal their identities." That was a kick in the stomach. So much for trying to break the silence surrounding epilepsy.

Dressed in a purple shirt, I went to all the schools and nurseries in my neighborhood and gave them the flyers I'd made. A few months later, in November, I arranged for a neurologist to speak to students and teachers to educate them about epilepsy since November is Epilepsy Awareness Month. However, the schools were pressed for time because of exams and the Palestine National Day celebration when schools had activities and events. It was too late to fit me in now but wanted me to come back in a few months. I preferred to wait until the following year and hold the event in November for Epilepsy Awareness Month. I wasn't discouraged by this initial rejection; if anything, I was more determined than ever.

Some of the schools asked me to talk, instead of the neurologist, since I had experienced living with epilepsy, but since public speaking isn't my strong suit, I declined. I planned to relaunch my epilepsy awareness campaign next year in November, and as part of that, I will make a short home video and talk about the stigma and shame many with epilepsy experience. Maybe it won't be as effective as speaking in schools, but perhaps it will give hope and strength to others suffering from epilepsy.

A year later, in January 2020, the Eyal Epilepsy Association invited me to join them at a conference in Tel Aviv. At their request, I brought along some of my flyers to distribute at the conference. This event was the first time I met the whole Eyal team in person, including Ophir. When we shook hands, happy tears filled my eyes; to my surprise, the same happened to him. It was a moment of joy and empathy.

Soon after, the association planned an event for Purple Day in 2020 at Hadassah Ein Karem Hospital where I had my surgery. They were going to set up a booth at the hospital, be available to answer any questions people may have had and try to educate anyone interested in learning more about epilepsy. However, the worldwide COVID-19 pandemic that started spreading made such events impossible, and it was canceled.

One of my biggest goals through all of this was to end the stigma surrounding epilepsy in Jerusalem. Living in a divided city like Jerusalem, where politics affects everything, it's never mattered to me if someone is Palestinian or Israeli. I just want the stigma to go away. Even though we as Palestinians struggle against Israeli military occupation, I want to break the silence surrounding epilepsy for everyone. It's not about Palestine and Israel; it's about a good cause: epilepsy.

After the conference, the Eyal Association called to ask if they could give my number to two different women in Gaza, Palestine. One was a teacher, and the other wanted to know more about the surgery I'd undergone. They both only spoke Arabic.

The teacher wanted to ask about a girl in her classroom

who would sometimes go blank and just stare straight ahead, with no movement. She wanted to know what to do when that happened. I told her that these types of seizures are known as 'absence seizures' and are very common in children. An absence seizure is a sudden brief lapse of consciousness, usually lasting under thirty seconds. The child appears to simply stare blankly for a few seconds. They may not even remember what happened, and they'll instantly return to being alert as soon as the seizure ends. Unfortunately, this affects their learning, and if a teacher doesn't know about it, they likely think the child is daydreaming or not paying attention. I explained to her that generally, there is no first aid needed for this type of seizure; she should just reassure the girl if she's frightened or upset by the experience. I also informed her about other types of seizures, such as complex-partial and grand mal seizures, and the first aid for them.

The other lady wanted to know about my surgery. She asked what my life was like while fighting epilepsy and how it changed for the better after surgery. She wanted to know if surgery was worth it, so I shared what I could. Halfway into our conversation, I could tell that she really wanted me to assure her that everything would be okay, which, of course, I couldn't do. Instead, I told her that I put my faith in the hands of God and prayed to St. Mar Charbel to be with me during my surgery.

That's when she told me that she was Muslim. Suddenly, I remembered a friend telling me about a prayer in Islam called an '*istikhara*,' in which a person asks God for help in a specific matter. So, I said to her, "Maybe the *istikhara* prayer would help you make your decision, because I can't make that decision for you."

She said, "How could I have ever forgotten about that

prayer? Thank you so much for reminding me! I'll do just that."

I always encourage people to consider undergoing the surgery and to be brave, but I could never tell them to do it. They must make that choice for themselves, often with God's help.

Chapter Thirty-Three

At the end of 2018, I decided it was time for me to look into having a bunionectomy, a surgical procedure to remove a bunion. A bunion is an enlargement of bone or soft tissues around the joint at the base of the big toe that results in the formation of a bump. As I got older, the bunions on both my feet started to hurt whenever I wore closed shoes, as the bunions would rub painfully when I walked. I've thought about having this surgery for years, but with my seizures, it seemed like too much to handle. It would've also been an extra load on Dimitri and the boys, which is the last thing I would've wanted. The orthopedic specialist recommended that I do both feet at the same time. This seemed wise; I might as well endure everything once. Plus, if I were to do each one separately, I might end up backing out of the second foot. This surgery is known to be very painful, but I figured that if I could survive the pain of brain surgery, I could survive the pain of this.

I completed all the necessary pre-surgery tests by the end of January 2019, and once again with the kind help of Dr. Basem, my surgery was scheduled for a week later, on the 5th of February, 2019, rather than mid-May.

because we lived in a hotel. However, I wish I'd given it more thought when I moved into a villa in Qatar or after I got married.

For years, my boys asked to get a dog. I always told them that when they were able to take care of it, we could get one. A few years after my surgery, Dimitri and the boys finally ganged up on me. The boys kept nagging, as kids do, and Dimitri cheered them on. They even got my mom involved; they knew she'd do everything in her power to convince me and she did. Finally, I gave in.

We started looking for a dog in 2020, and it was a surprising difficult search. There were no pets available anywhere because the COVID-19 pandemic was in full swing, and according to the pet shops we'd visited, everyone was buying a pet during that time. One pet store told us that they could pre-order a golden retriever puppy for us, and when a mother gave birth, they'd get one of her puppies for us. The boys didn't want to wait, though; they were too excited. We kept looking and finally found a Yorkshire Terrier. We brought her home and named her Brooklyn.

We told the boys that they now had to keep their word and take care of her. That went well for the first two or three days, but after that, they wanted to go out and have fun with their friends, too. Taking care of the dog wasn't always their first priority.

At first, Brooklyn and I kept our distance. I wasn't used to having a pet, and I wasn't ready yet to pet her, hold her, or have her sit beside me. When we were in the same room, she'd either be sitting in her bed or on the couch across from me. Eventually, she would get closer and closer until she was sitting right next to me. She won my heart in the end, and she continues to hold it to this day.

At night, she usually sleeps in the boys' room. We have an open-door policy at home, but after we got Brooklyn, I started to shut my bedroom door at night. I wasn't used to that, but I didn't want Brooklyn sleeping in my room, as I still wasn't used to her or fully comfortable around her. It got to the point where, as soon as I closed the door, she'd come stand outside it. Sometimes, when I went into my room at night to go to sleep, I'd find her lying on my side of my bed, right beneath my pillow, and I'd ask the boys to take her out. They both finally said, "Do you want her to hate us? She wants to be with you! You take her out." One night, she appeared to be fast asleep, and I couldn't bring myself to wake her, so I finally left the door open. She soon began to make herself comfy at the foot of our bed each night. Now, she makes herself comfortable wherever she likes and practically owns the bed.

It's hard not to spoil Brooklyn. I have become very attached to her. When we travel for long periods of time, she travels with us. My cousins and friends always tease me about how much I love her because I constantly have something to say about her. So, to pick on me and have a laugh, they'll purposely ask about her, knowing that I'll go on and on about her.

One of my classmates in Bahrain, Heidi, recently passed away during her battle with cancer. We were in touch through Facebook, and we used to share our poetry, since she loved writing poems, too. When I learned of her death, my tears were unstoppable, so I got up and dimmed the lights so no one would see me. A short while later, I saw Brooklyn making her way toward me. She had been sleeping on our bed. She sat down beside me in her own cute way and gave me some emotional comfort. If I had gotten a dog when I had epilepsy, it definitely would have helped with my seizures, my emotional distress, and my mental health.

Chapter Thirty-Four

I have now been completely seizure free for 7 years. My five-year seizure free anniversary called for a celebration, but it came during the pandemic, so everyone was couped up at home and nothing was open. Nadine still wanted to make it special and not let it pass just like any other day, though, so she decided to make a video to congratulate me on passing this milestone. She had all my family and friends from all over the world record short messages for me. With Samar's video making expertise, she helped put all these clips together, added photos from the time of my surgery and amazing background music, and turned it into the most amazing heartfelt thirty-minute video. I cried continuously while watching it. It meant the world to me, and I will cherish it forever.

After I watched this, I sent out the emotional thank-you message I mentioned earlier, that I thought would make the normally stoic Lorine cry.

Life with my new brain has been magnificent, but there's always that fear that my seizures will return. Studies suggest that if you do not have a seizure in the first year after temporal lobe surgery—with medication—the likelihood of being seizure free at the two-year mark is 87–90 percent. If you have not had a seizure in two years, the likelihood of being seizure free is 95 percent at five years and 82 percent at ten years. After one year without seizures, your doctor may consider tapering off your anti-epileptic medication and eventually taking you off the drugs entirely. Most people who do experience a seizure after going off medication are able to control them again entirely by resuming the medication. I have continued taking medicine since my surgery; I don't want to get off it. I'd rather be on the safe side. Dr. Dana agrees with me, though now, I'm only taking Lamictal.

A year after my surgery, in October 2016, I started to gradually reduce my dosage of Levetiracetam, the generic form of Keppra, and in January of 2017, I was completely free of it. At that time, I was still taking 1500 milligrams of Lamictal per day. Once I had been off the Levetiracetam for six months, I started gradually reducing my Lamictal dosage as well. By mid-2018, I was down to 250 milligrams of Lamictal twice a day. I've been on that dosage ever since. For seizure medication, this is considered an extremely low dosage.

Lamictal has the fewest side effects of all the anti-epileptic medications I've taken over the years. It does cause blurred vision, double vision, poor coordination, depression, and anxiety, but it doesn't severely affect my mental health the way Levetiracetam, Topamax, and all the other medications I used to take did. In addition, since my seizures themselves also caused behavioral problems, just being seizure free has greatly improved my mental health.

It's wonderful to be able to master and nurture my mind. I now have the power to control my thoughts, moods, and behavior. I can create balance, keep my mind calm, and feed it with positive thoughts. I am free of mental slavery. I now have the freedom to make choices about my health and medications. In countless ways, this surgery was the best thing to ever happen to me.

I've had numerous MRIs and EEGs over the past seven years, and there is absolutely no sign that my seizures will return. But one day three-and-a-half years after my surgery, when I had just reached the reduction stage of Lamictal to 250 milligrams twice daily, I felt something that I have always associated with having a seizure but might not have anything to do with epilepsy at all. It was like the feelings that used to descend before I had an aura. For a moment, all I could think about was that I was about to have another seizure. But then, I didn't have an aura. I didn't lose consciousness or control of my body. So, I got in touch with Dr. Dana and underwent an MRI and EEG. There was no sign of epileptic activity. I was incredibly relieved.

Then, about six months later, it happened again. I tried to remain positive and not let it get to me. After all, the last thing I want is to live in fear of having another seizure.

Sometime in 2019, it happened again, so I sent Rebbeca a message and asked her to schedule an appointment for me with Dr. Dana. I wanted to ask her if she could write me a referral for another EEG and MRI. Rebbeca called me so we could discuss what was happening and why I felt I needed to repeat those tests. Since my 2018 test results showed no sign of epileptic activity, she felt it wasn't necessary to do them again and suggested it might be psychological. I was surprised by her assumption; after all, I'm the only one who could judge whether these sensations were psychological or physical because I was the one experiencing them. On the other hand, I understood why she would say that. All she had to go off was the medical test results, so I didn't take offense. On the contrary, I would much rather have the issue be psychological—or anything else for that matter—than it be a return of my seizures.

Still, I was determined to find out why I was experiencing these sensations, since my previous tests indicated that nothing was wrong with me. I started doing extensive research on many different websites. When I first experienced this in mid-2018, I jotted down the details of what happened and what I had been doing at the time. If it was a seizure, I wanted to be able to pinpoint the responsible trigger. As it turned out, in doing so, I was able to find the most likely explanation for what was happening to me.

I now believe that I was experiencing a panic attack and that it will never turn into a seizure. Panic attacks occur suddenly and without warning, so they are extremely frightening. A panic attack is a sudden surge of intense fear or anxiety that may or may not have a known cause or is disproportionate to the perceived threat. This intense fear comes with some psychological symptoms as well as physical symptoms that are similar to a heart attack or the beginning of a seizure. A panic attack can last anywhere from several seconds to several minutes.

When I still had seizures, I would often feel anxious, overwhelmed, or fearful before having an aura. I now believe that I was often having panic attacks before having a seizure and that these feelings were not at all associated with my epilepsy.

I also learned that Lamictal is not only used to control seizures but also to help with anxiety. However, some individuals may not respond well to the neurochemical modulation induced by Lamictal and may experience heightened anxiety instead. Taking 1500 milligrams of Lamictal helped with my anxiety symptoms. However, now that I was taking only 500 milligrams of Lamictal a day, this dosage wasn't enough to prevent me from having these rare panic attacks.

According to Epilepsy Action, the symptoms of anxiety, particularly panic attacks, can look and feel a lot like the symptoms of some epileptic seizures. This means that both conditions can be misdiagnosed. However, since the surgery was a success for me and these feelings only started in mid-2018 when I had reached a low dosage of Lamictal, I chose to believe that I was experiencing the occasional panic attack, not symptoms related to epilepsy.

As an example, one time, Dimitri, Johnny, and I were walking around Dubai Mall, the largest mall in the world. We were on the third floor, which is already very high up. There was a newly built escalator that went up an additional floor above the third and led to a small, high, secluded, glass-covered terrace. Johnny wanted to go up and see it, so he asked me to go up with him. I didn't feel comfortable going up, but he insisted and ran off toward it. Watching him going up the escalator, I felt an intense fear of losing control. Difference Between.net best describes what I felt. It's a sense of impending doom that settled over me. At the same time, my heart rate increased, and I began to hyperventilate. My mind raced, and I felt on edge. This all happened in a matter of seconds. It was caused by my subconscious mind worrying about the worst-case scenarios: "What if he leans over the bars and falls down? What if the bars he's leaning on break? I should've gone with him, just in case." It was all happening too fast, and then, within seconds, the panic was over.

I realized that Rebbeca was somewhat correct in her initial assessment, and I sent her a message letting her know that.

These panic attacks are difficult to ignore or move past right away because they end up worrying me for a while afterward, but I can live with them because they're very rare and are not related to my seizures.

My last follow-up MRI and EEG were done at the end of 2021, and there was still no sign of epileptic activity. That said, Dr. Dana did tell me that these tests might not be able to track very brief epileptic events that occur at irregular intervals.

If my seizures ever do come back, I'd be outraged, but I have absolutely no regrets about having had the surgery. It allowed me to take control of my life. I also believe that if, God forbid, my seizures ever do return, they won't be as bad as they were before—frequent and severe. I feel certain that the Lamictal medication is what's controlling them and preventing them from happening. And, as strange as it may sound, if the worst were to happen, I'd just have another surgery.

Chapter Thirty-Five

The years I have spent being seizure free have been the best years of my life. If I ever have to live with epilepsy again, I'll use everything I've learned during this time to maintain my positive outlook way of life. I'll never forget how blessed I was during my twenty-five-year journey to have such caring, supportive family and friends in my life. I am and will forever be grateful to them. Still, there's nothing that compares with experiencing freedom at its fullest—the feeling of being free to pick up and go where I want, when I want, without having to plan and worry and think in advance about all the things that could go wrong. I love having complete control over myself and my mind and not having a care in the world for the trivial things that used to hold me back. I can simply live in the present moment. Everyone who knew me during my journey—my mood swings, my temper, my unstable personality—has seen a drastic change in me, and they have pointed it out because it's so noticeable and real.

The first thing I did was pull the boys off the school bus and start driving them to and from school again. I also started taking Anya and her sister Suzi with us since they're

sports academy. The coaches were brought in from Spain. In 2018, when Joseph was eleven years old, the academy arranged for a ten-day program for the kids to go visit the main academy in Spain and train with the coaches there. Joseph traveled to Barcelona with his teammates, and we went along as well, since it was his first time to be alone away from home. Plus, we didn't want Johnny to feel left out, since the training camp was during their Easter break. Many other parents traveled with their kids as well, and this was the first time I got to meet some of the moms and dads and feel involved in Joseph's after school activity.

A few months after the Barcelona trip, Johnny started going to football practice with Joseph, too. But now, I was the one driving them, as I'd just bought a car. I also took two other boys who lived in our neighborhood. Joseph and Johnny would sometimes come up to me during practice when they needed something. They were thrilled that I was present during their practices, and I loved being there, too. I also met so many wonderful moms at practice. I already knew some of them because their boys also attended JAS, but there were many other moms whose children attended other schools. Making friends has never been a problem for me, but being seizure free made it easier to want to be social and connect with people; I no longer had to worry about having a seizure or making a bad impression because of my unpredictable behavior and uncontrolled mood swings. I was my real self.

Sometimes, the moms would go on a walk on a trail right beside the football field. When I started attending practices, one of the moms asked me if I'd like to join them on their walks, and so I did. We would watch our boys for a while, then go for a walk.

During the winter, we'd all freeze while sitting on the bleachers, wearing beanies and holding our to-go mugs of coffee, but it was fun chatting and bonding. I would never have been able to do that prior to my surgery, because getting cold was a trigger for my seizures. One time at practice, it was just too cold, so we all squeezed into two cars parked beside each other in the parking lot, opened the windows halfway, and chatted. We simply made the best out of it.

Just being present like the other moms was enough for my boys, regardless of whether I went for a walk or sat on the bleachers throughout practice and watched them play. For me, seeing the happiness in their eyes now that I was more involved in their lives was the greatest satisfaction of all.

I was confused and caught off-guard by her reactions. Why would she say such a thing? I had never spoken to her before today.

But apparently, that wasn't true. Areen had approached me many years ago at Sunshine Nursery while picking up Zein. Little did I know that Zein and Johnny had been classmates since nursery, before they both moved to JAS. Back then, she had once asked me if I'd like to plan a play-date for our boys. My reaction was, in her words, "You gave me a faint smile, like, 'Okay, whatever,' and walked off. I thought you were so full of yourself and extremely rude."

I wasn't at all shocked to hear what her first impression of me had been because, at that exact time, my life had just been turned upside down again. I had just recently stopped driving, so I was very depressed and just wanted to be left alone. I was still meeting with people I knew, but I didn't want to make other friends or interact with anyone new. I knew people wouldn't understand me, and I didn't have the positive energy to put any effort into forging a new social life. I already had enough friends who knew me for who I really am and who I was still very much in contact with, so at the time, I preferred to keep to myself and to my circle of friends.

Today, I occasionally tease Areen about her first impression of me when we get together. By now, she knows that she'll never hear the end of it.

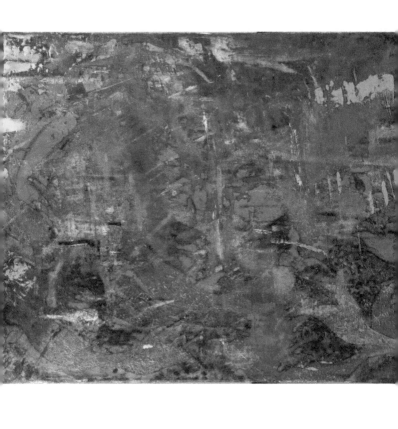

Sixth Sense

Look at me from a distance
and you will see
painted brush strokes
splashed on canvas freely
An interpretation of a painting
that's been seen by the naked eye
a hasty assumption
that's been thoroughly criticized

Look at me closely
and you will see
character sketch scribbles
splashed on canvas in disguise

An impression of a painting
that meets the naked eye
a false perception
that's been partially analyzed

Approach me without judgment
and let your instinct decide
is it friendly mermaids flapping their tails
or sly sneaky foxes with more than one face

Even though I've never been allowed to travel alone, I've long been familiar with the various airport formalities and travel procedures. I've always been the one who takes care of the flight bookings, visas, and packing, and during the pandemic, I took care of all the COVID-19 paperwork and travel regulations. Even after my surgery, we continued to always travel as a family. There's just no reason for me to travel alone.

The single exception occurred six years after my surgery, when we were all going to visit my parents in Dubai for Christmas. A week before our flight, Dimitri discovered that he'd have to fly out to Dubai on business earlier than we had planned. Since Joseph and Johnny still had midterms, we couldn't leave earlier with him. But for the first time, there was no need to panic or figure things out. Dimitri left early, and everything else went as previously planned. I was able to do everything I needed to do; there was no need for anyone to worry about me being home alone with the boys or having to take care of us. A week later, the boys and I met up with Dimitri in Dubai.

The following summer, Samar got married and asked me if I would be her bridesmaid. It was such an honor to be part of her bridal party. Being seizure free made it very possible for me to accept Samar's request without hesitation and not have to turn her down as I would've had to if I was still having seizures. As foolish as that may sound, considering she's like my little sister and I hold so much love for her, my withdrawal would've only been for her sake. After all, there would have been a high probability that I have a seizure, make a scene walking ahead of her, and potentially ruin her walk down the aisle.

I still go to my aunt and uncle's house to see them while the boys are at school most days of the week, as I used to. They are very important to me, and I love to see them any chance I get. Just because they no longer need to take care of me and I can now get things done on my own, it doesn't mean I don't make time to see them.

It is and always has been very important to me to appreciate the people who have helped me. I've always loved helping people too. It makes me feel happy to see people happy. Some may call this being a people-pleaser; I call it kindness. Kindness comes from within. It's giving without expectation of reward. I don't need a reason to do it. I do it because it feels good to give and not just take in life. I will never forget anything anyone has done for me, and I will be forever grateful for it. During my journey, I have always done my best to give back. Epilepsy affected everyone in my life; my family and friends spent so much time and effort doing things for me that I couldn't do on my own. Just because they made it seem effortless, it doesn't mean that it was. Regardless of how miserable or hopeless I felt during my battle with epilepsy, even when I was at my lowest, showing my gratitude made me feel whole. Being there for others and helping when I could brought me enormous satisfaction. Look beyond yourself and count your blessings every single day; you'll be amazed at what life gives back.

A few days before Joseph's teacher went back to the US for good, I invited her over for dinner to bid her farewell. She had been his homeroom teacher during the time of my surgery and had done so much to support him. We talked all night about so many different things, including my journey with epilepsy. About half an hour before she left, she said to me, "With everything you've been through, it's amazing how many times you've thanked God for your blessings while talking about your battle with epilepsy."

I appreciate my mom and dad, Nadine, Dimitri, Joseph, Johnny, all my extended family, and my friends tremendously. I would go to the ends of the earth for them. But

perfectly in that issue, which was focused on social responsibility.

Once again, several schools asked me to talk to their students and share my personal experiences with epilepsy. However, as much as I wanted to do that, I still couldn't. So, I finally took the plunge and made the video that I'd been thinking about since my first attempt at an awareness campaign a few years ago. It was short and straight to the point, with no medical terminology so students wouldn't get bored and lose interest. Maybe one day I'll find the courage to stand in front of a crowd and share my experiences, but not yet.

Joseph and Johnny continue to express their happiness about the success of my surgery and the fact that I no longer suffer from seizures. They are proud to share this information with their friends. Both are now taller than me and turning into wonderful young men whom I'll always be proud of. I love them with all my heart. They will forever be my heroes and most precious treasures.

Sometimes only after the fact do you realize the huge impact of something you thought was small at the time. Johnny was in seventh grade during the epilepsy campaign I launched in 2021. He repeatedly told me how proud he was of me and wanted nothing more than for me to tell my story to his school, especially in front of his classmates. Johnny wanted people to know that I was the one behind the epilepsy awareness campaign. He once said to me, "People should know that you're the one doing all these things, because you deserve the credit." I told him that the whole purpose of the campaign is to educate people. It's not about who gets the credit. I later found out that he was telling some of his friends that I'm writing a book about my journey with epilepsy. I saw the mom of Johnny's friend, Amir, at school and she asked about my book. Surprised, I said to her "how did you know I was writing a book?" she said, "Johnny told Amir about it."

At this point, neither of the boys had seen the video I made, and Johnny refused to watch it except with his classmates. My video talks about how my seizures started, how to help someone who is having a seizure, how my family and others helped me, how I handled it, what I've accomplished during my journey, and what I learned from living with seizures. I suddenly realized that my boys only know what they witnessed and nothing more. Almost 75 percent of what I said on the video, they'd never heard before. We had never discussed these things before; they never came up in conversation. After all, why would I want to raise the issue after the fact and remind them of unpleasant memories from the past?

Even though I targeted my video toward high school students, Johnny's teachers and educational *counselor* did everything in their power to find the time to play it in front of Johnny's seventh-grade classmates, making his wishes come true. Some of the teachers already knew the impact my surgery had on him, so they knew how important this was to him. He was so excited when he found out that my video was going to be played during an assembly in front of all the seventh graders together and not separately during homeroom, as originally planned. He even asked the assistant principal for upper elementary to introduce the video by saying that this video was about Johnny's mom, just to make sure his classmates would pay attention.

Apparently, on the day of the assembly, Johnny also asked her if he could say a few words after the video ended, and she kindly agreed. He told his classmates about a time when I had a seizure and what he did to help. Based on his actions throughout this campaign, I believe that it gave him closure. It was his own way of letting go of the past. Not

received a phone call from Joyce. She said, "I wanted to talk to you about the epilepsy campaign you carried out in November and express my gratitude for your effort and initiative in bringing awareness to such an important medical disorder that is ignored in our society."

I guess word travels fast in our community; I didn't know she knew that I was behind it. I thanked her for the compliment and thought that was the end of it, but it wasn't.

She continued, "I want to share something with you that happened as a result of your campaign. I was visiting my brother, and we were talking about Tina's disorder and how things were going with her. His kids were playing nearby. You know how kids are: when you call for them, they don't listen, and when you're carrying on a conversation with someone else, their ears are like radar antennae. My nephew said to us from behind, 'You're talking about epilepsy' and both our jaws dropped. We knew we were talking about epilepsy, but how did he? I said, 'How do you know what we're talking about?' and he said, 'I learned about it in class from my teacher. From what you're describing, Tina definitely has epilepsy.' We were taken by surprise because we didn't expect that coming from a sixth grader. It was impressive that he was aware of it because it really is important. He now knows what is happening to Tina and understands that it's a disorder. I salute you and thank you for that. I always thank God for that day at the club when you shared your epilepsy disorder with me and for the day I saw you at the wedding reception. God works in such mysterious ways to bring us together just around the time Tina started to show symptoms so I could ask you about them and so you could guide me. You truly are a godsend. I also wanted to ask if Tina can watch the video you made so she knows she's not alone."

My mind was blown hearing this story. I was so happy, I felt as if I were bouncing off the walls. My awareness campaign really was effective and got students' and teachers' attention.

Joyce's nephew was a student at JAS. So, the next day, I called the communications coordinator who helped me organize the event at JAS and shared this amazing news with her. I thanked her for all her efforts and the teachers' efforts in making this possible. She was as blown away as I was. I also asked her to share this story with the teachers so they would know how appreciated they are and how critical their dedication to teaching is. My goal with this campaign has always been to reach as many people as possible and to encourage local institutions to continue the momentum and support this cause on an annual basis.

Living with epilepsy has made me stronger, braver, more understanding, and kinder. It taught me to appreciate people more. Your power lies within you. Honor your resilience and courage in the face of adversity. As Dennis Kimbro says, "Life is 10% what happens to us and 90% how we react to it."

This is the painting and its poem which I had referred to in chapter 25. They were created after I became seizure free and illustrate a huge change in color and tone.

Acknowledgments

There are many people who helped bring this book to completion and I would like to express my deepest gratitude to each of them. The experience of writing a memoir is both internally challenging and rewarding.

To my precious family who inspire me every day. I will eternally be indebted to you. Thank you for your encouragement and full support when I started writing this book. I couldn't have written it without you. I love you infinitely.

My admirable dad Johnny, my *idol*. Your love, care, protection, and phenomenal success in life has always given me courage to believe that I can achieve anything I put my mind to and not give up on life. You tried to move mountains for me, and my security was your greatest desire. You are truly an amazing man and father, and I'm so proud to be your daughter! Thank you for supporting my decision to have brain surgery. You have a heart as big as the ocean with tides full of inspiration, kindness, generosity, support, patience, wisdom, and a lifetime of eternal unconditional love that infinitely sway my way. For all that you are and all that you do, there aren't enough words to express the love I hold for you. Thank you for giving me everything and for helping me to get to where I am today.

My one-of-a-kind mom, Norma my *savior*. You share the purest love, filled my life with happiness, comfort, wisdom, strength, care, and guidance. You've made so many sacri-

My heartfelt appreciation and gratitude go to my extended family members in Jerusalem: Anisa Kreitem, Salwa Zananiri, Janet Jawharieh, Antoinette Diliani, Samar Zananiri, Soula Kreitem, Marwa Kreitem, Lorine Shubeitah, Dima Rofa and to your spouses. Your presence, unconditional love, kindness, and unparalleled support were a vital part in my journey. You stood by me during my struggles and accepted my behavioral patterns. Thank you for everything you have done for me. I'll forever be grateful to you for lending me a helping hand when I needed it and I am extremely blessed to have been surrounded by you all. Thank you for taking care of my boys during my stay at the hospital, after surgery, and during my recovery period. I love each one of you with all my heart.

To Nada Kazimi, Nisreen Salem, and Lama Zeidan: you were an essential part of my daily life during my entire journey, and I am forever thankful to you. You each helped me survive my sorrows through many difficult times. You never judged me, and you stood by me no matter the circumstance. You always gave me an encouraging word, helped me see the good in everything and brought love and joy into my life. You are with whom I can be the truest version of myself. Thank you for your true genuine friendship and for bearing my burdens. I will forever treasure our sweet memories and exciting adventures. I'm so lucky we're still making more memories together, but now with our families and children. You will always hold a very special place in my heart.

To Lara Manougian, Lina Hashem, Fatima Javed, Kerry Walker, and Rasha El-Shurafa: your friendship is very precious and rare. No matter how much time passes, when we do meet up it's as if we saw each other yesterday. I will always cherish the great memories we shared which always make me smile, the amazing adventures we had and to know that my friendship with you will last forever. Thank you for being there for me when my life turned upside down, for sharing happiness and laughter, kindness and care, and for always being by my side when I needed you most. I am so lucky to have friends like you in my life. You mean so much to me, more than you'll ever know.

To Munia Awan: you saw my potential from the very beginning which encouraged me to excel and gave me the confidence to dream big. To Dr. Imad Kanaan, Dr. Dana, Ekstein, and Dr. Moni Benifla: you gave me first-class medical treatment and valuable advice which resulted in setting me free of my seizures. To Jeffrey Goldstein: you helped me strengthen my healing vortex and brought to light my true self. To Dr. Basem Abuasab: thank you for your continued support in fundraising my epilepsy awareness campaigns in Jerusalem. To the Jerusalem American School faculty: your understanding, patience, and compassion towards my boys during difficult times was exemplary. Thank you all, I will forever cherish you.

I would like to extend my sincere appreciation to Jeanne Boles, Rinal Abu Shanab, Nibal Karkar, and Nelima Lassen for sharing your experiences in my book. I also want to thank everyone I've mentioned within my chapters along with countless others who have helped me along the way.

———————

I praise and thank God, every day, for getting me through all the challenges I've faced, answering my prayers, and granting me countless blessings. I will always have faith in you.

References

Epilepsy Foundation - *Unwavering Ally on a Journey with Epilepsy and Seizures* https://www.epilepsy.com/

WHO World Health Organization - *Key Facts About Epilepsy*
https://www.who.int/news-room/fact-sheets/detail/epilepsy

MECPsych – *Factors Affecting Stigma of Epilepsy*
https://journals.lww.com/mecpsychiatry/fulltext/2017/07000/Factors_affecting_stigma_of_epilepsy.4.aspx

Single Care - *Topamax Side Effects and how to Avoid Them*
https://www.singlecare.com/blog/topamax-side-effects/

Eyal Epilepsy Association – Website I volunteered for and wrote their English content
https://www.epilepsy.org.il

Sunrise Ranch - *What is Attunement?* www.sunriseranch.org/attunement

Fractual Enlightenment - *Understanding Brainwaves to Expand our Consciousness*
https://fractalenlightenment.com/14794/spirituality/understanding-braiwaves-to-expand-our-consciousness

Pacific College of Health and Science - *Benefits of TCM and Acupuncture for Epilepsy*
https://www.pacificcollege.edu/news/blog/2015/01/18/the-benefits-of-tcm-and-acupuncture-for-epilepsy

MedicineNet - *What is an Amygdalohippocampectomy, its Risks and Complications*
https://www.medicinenet.com/risks_complications_amygdalohippocampectomy/article.htm

9 781637 7733

Kaya's Journey

A Legend of Kaya Novel

Ashley Marie Spencer

Prologue

"Alright, you ready for round two?" Kiyahe asked me from behind the camera as I returned to my perch on the hard, wooden stool for the second day in a row.

Yesterday I had re-told my tale of how I'd survived a horrendous apocalyptic disaster, lost everything I cared about, travelled hundreds of miles on foot, and discovered my new family and my new purpose.

It was exhausting just to think about all I'd been through, let alone to have lived it.

I rolled my eyes at Kiyahe, whose attention was focused on attaching the bulky, black contraption to its tripod. It didn't matter whether I was ready, I had to get this done. Why did he even bother asking? I was never *ready* for what I had to do anyways. My life had been speeding ahead of my brain and my heart for a long while now, like a racecar on a speedway. It was all I could do to not look like a drunk driver behind the wheel.

Instead of responding to his rhetorical question with something snarky, as I usually did, I bit my tongue and concentrated on the blinking red light that would glow steadily once we started filming.

I fidgeted with my finger nails, trying to pick the dirt out from under them. At least the one's that weren't chewed down to the quick anyway. Speaking in front of people made me nervous and it was all I could do to keep from chewing my fingers right off. Granted, I wasn't speaking to *people*, necessarily, I was speaking to a camera. But I had to *imagine* I was speaking to people.

My people.

Kiyahe noticed my uncharacteristic silence and turned his brilliant blue eyes on me, a look of concern and sympathy plain on his features. My breath caught and my heart stuttered, it was impossible to think, impossible to *focus* when both of us had our guards down at the same time. Suddenly I didn't care about making a documentary for future generations. All I wanted was for him to take me away and hold me. To tell me someone else would take care of everything, that I didn't have to be in charge anymore.

But that would be a lie and Kiyahe never lied to me.

I waved my hand dismissively before he could ask me what was wrong and tried to put on a brave smile for him. It felt more like a warped grimace.

Today I would have to tell the camera and future generations about my journey across the country with Kiyahe, Neka, and Shilah as we'd attempted to unite the remaining tribes and their people into a new nation. It was going to be harder to talk about this journey than the one I'd travelled on my own. My first journey from South Dakota to Oklahoma after the meteor shower disaster, or the Fire Rains as the people called it, was easier for me to talk about because I had been responsible for only myself and no one else. Plus, I had had to tell that story dozens of times to each tribe we'd met along the second journey.

On my second, more arduous journey, I had been responsible for winning over thousands of people and convincing them that our survival depended on us becoming one people, with only my word and their faith to back it up. I had made friends, I had made enemies, I had made alliances, and I had made messes.

Dozens of times I had tried to tell God or the Great Spirit or whoever was running the show that I was not cut out for this. Someone had cast a chorus girl as the lead role and she had no idea what the hell she was doing.

But the show must go on, right?

So instead of getting off the stool and running from the room, which I verily wanted to do, I squared my shoulders and straightened my spine. While Kiyahe switched out the tapes in the dinosaur of a camera that we were using and adjusted the camera settings, I focused on trying to look like the noble leader everyone wanted me to be. I raised my chin, narrowed my eyes, and planted my gaze firmly on the blinking red light on top of the camera.

I must have looked as ridiculous as I felt because when Kiyahe glanced up from adjusting the tripod base, his eyebrows scrunched in confusion.

"What the hell are you doing?" he asked. "You're going to break the camera staring at it like that."

My poor attempt at looking noble slid off my face and a flush of embarrassment replaced it. I stuttered and mumbled, "Nothing, I... I just... don't worry about it, alright? Just get the damn camera ready."

When Kiyahe was all set, I clasped my hands tightly in my lap to keep from fidgeting. He gave me the same advice as yesterday, trying to calm my nerves and ease me into the memories of our second journey.

"Now just relax, Marie. Do like you did yesterday and just tell the next part of the story like you're telling it to me. If we can get it right the first time, we can be done for the day."

I nodded and closed my eyes, thinking back through the memories of all that had transpired on our road trip across the country. All the tribes we had visited. All the people we had met. Each memory flickering behind my eyelids in time with my heartbeat. My subconscious registered that Kiyahe's breathing had matched my own and that our syncopation was the only sound in the room. I wondered if he was thinking back on it all too.

I opened my stormy, grey-blue eyes and looked into his bright turquoise one's across the room. He was watching and waiting for me to give him the signal to start recording.

I felt a swell of happiness that Kiyahe was my life-bound protector. With him by my side, sometimes I really did feel like I could do anything. He was always telling me to be myself. Reminding me that my down-to-earth, honest, humble, and loyal personality was what drew the people to me. What convinced them that I would be a good leader. So instead of putting on a face and pretending to be something I wasn't, I told the next part of our story in the only way I knew how.

I started where I had left off.

The strength to be strong enough not to be weak. The courage to be tall enough not to be small. The clear vision to see where I've been. The guidance to take me where I'm going.

—Haida Prayer.

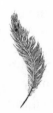

Chapter One

"How much longer til we get there? My God, Shilah, you are the slowest driver in the world!"

Neka sighed dramatically and rolled over on the couch so that he was on his stomach and his face was buried in a throw pillow. His muffled complaints continued while Kiyahe and I stared vacantly out the windows of the bus and while Shilah shouted back from the driver's seat.

"I'm going as fast as I can with all these craters and piles of cement in the way, you pain in the ass! I'd like to see you try to drive through all this crap!"

Neka rolled again so that his face was free of the pillow and Shilah could hear him clearly.

"I could! And I could do it in half the time that it's taking you!"

"Half drowned rat!"

"Tub of lard!"

"SHUT UP!" Kiyahe and I yelled at the same time. Kiyahe and I looked at each other in surprise before looking away hastily. Neka glanced back and forth between us before shoving his face back into the throw pillow. Shilah glowered at the windshield. Everyone was silent then.

The twins had been bickering almost the entire drive so far. But part of me couldn't blame them, at least it was something to *do*. We'd been on the road for hours as we made our way from Oklahoma to Texas and still had several more hours to go. Our trek was being dragged out

a squashed bug on the outside of my window. We'd been doing this for hours. Sneaking glances at each other when we thought the other wouldn't notice. Saying nothing.

When Kiyahe's eyes went back to the map, I turned and looked behind me at Neka, who stared at the ceiling in boredom as he laid on the couch next to Kiyahe's chair. He had claimed that couch as his to sleep on while Shilah had claimed the one across from it, the currently empty one that was next to the booth where I was sitting. There was a bunk room with three bunks on each side of the wall, past a door behind the main room where we were sitting now. The twins had insisted the bunks were too hard to sleep on and that it would be better if someone were sleeping in the room where the bus door was, in case someone tried to come in the bus while we were parked at night.

Kiyahe would sleep in the bunk room alone then. A door led from the bunk room to the very back room in the bus, my bedroom. As my life-long, soul-bound, primary protector, he insisted that he sleep nearest to me for my protection. And although we had slept in the same one-room tent together on our "bonding journey," he didn't offer to sleep that close to me again and I didn't ask him to. I was glad to know that even if he didn't like me, he still cared enough to protect me.

This sleeping arrangement was in case someone had the guts enough to try and get on the bus in the middle of the night to hurt me, which was highly unlikely. But as my protectors, the boys took their jobs seriously and wanted to be prepared for any possibility.

The more concerning issue regarding my protection wasn't what would happen while we were on the bus, but rather what would happen once we left it.

As we travelled from state-to-state, tribe-to-tribe, we would stick to a plan the boys had devised. We would park the bus in a concealed area at least a mile away from the tribe we were visiting. Then myself, Kiyahe, and one of the twins would walk to the tribe to give our spiel while the other of the twins would wait back at the bus. We would be impossibly outnumbered wherever we went, even if all four of us went together, so the boys had decided I would take as much protection as possible and whichever twin was left behind with the bus would be ready in case we had to make a run for it.

In case the tribe chased us out of town or tried to kill me.

In case they wouldn't listen.

In case I'd failed.

We would also go in armed with weapons from a large collection that we were carrying. I had brought my bow, and Kiyahe didn't want me to try and hide it, he wanted the people we met to know I could defend myself. Kiyahe and whichever of the twins went with us would carry hand guns concealed in secret holsters in their jackets. We didn't want to scare anyone, but we didn't want to feel as vulnerable as we were either.

As I ran through our planned procedures in my head and imagined the worst possible outcomes, I nearly missed the large sign on the side of the road that announced we'd crossed state borders.

"We're in Texas now ya'll!" Shilah twanged excitedly from the driver's seat up front. Neka rolled his eyes but sat up on his couch, more alert. Kiyahe tucked the map into his jacket and wiped his hands on his jeans before standing. Neka and I looked up at him expectantly and Shilah stopped humming up front so he could hear clearly.

"Ok, so the Comanche will be our first tribe and probably one of our largest. My father doubts that all the tribes we're visiting have survived the Fire Rains unscathed. Even so, they'll probably be much larger than our own tribe." Kiyahe spoke with reverence and determination, like an army general preparing his troops for their next mission. As much as he tended to irritate and confuse me, I listened with respect. Kiyahe had been educated as a chief's son which meant he knew better than the rest of us what to expect from the tribes we would encounter.

"Historically the Comanche were independent, tough, and strong. They were soldiers and fighters. Although they didn't go out looking for trouble, they had no problem fighting trouble off. My father thinks they will be tough but fair to us, guarded but open-minded."

The twins listened earnestly, Neka nodding his head as Kiyahe spoke, while I tried to fight back nausea. We were really doing this! And I had no idea what to do or say or how to behave! I swallowed back the bile that rose in my throat and blinked furiously against the forming moisture in my eyes. Why had I agreed to do something I had no idea how to do?!

"Excuse me," I mumbled as I lurched from the booth and powerwalked to my bedroom at the back of the bus, slamming the door behind me. I held my arms above my head, closed my eyes, and took deep breaths in through my nose and out through my mouth. I tried not to think about an entire race of people dying out if I failed.

Instead I directed my thoughts to the smell of my parent's house, the sound of my old boss, Julio's laugh, the simplicity of nature as I'd walked across it for hundreds of miles, the power of my bow when I shot it, the purity of my wolf's eyes, the sparkle of my new little sister, Hiawassee's smile, the warm hug of her mother, Mahala, and the sincerity of Kiyahe's turquoise gaze.

I was mentally lost in those eyes when a soft knock on the door startled me. I leaned my head against the paper-thin, veneer door but did not open it.

"I'm fine. Go away," I said as bravely as I could to the wood grain in front of my face.

"No, you're not, what's wrong?" Kiyahe asked softly from the other side.

I didn't answer, I just focused on my breathing.

He knew the answer, probably before he'd even asked the question.

"You can do this, Marie. We believe in you. You just have to believe in yourself."

My nostrils flared, I'd heard this speech from everyone a dozen times each. It didn't make things easier, it only made my weakness more infuriating.

I pulled back from the door and flung it open before shouting at him.

were far worse than this one behind the counter. The ones I had seen were fresh at first, the cause of death written plainly on their charred skin or blood-soaked lips. People who had burned to death from the fires the meteors had ignited or who had choked out their life's blood from inhaling all the smoke and debris kicked up by the blasts. Many people had also been killed by being crushed under the massive meteors or buried alive underneath them, but those bodies I hadn't had to see.

It had gotten worse as the days and weeks went by. The bodies had decomposed rapidly under the blistering sun and heat. But their rotting hadn't been fast enough to spare me the gruesome scenes. I could still remember the swelling and bloating of the bodies as they boiled. I could still remember the smell, the absolutely revolting scent as they rotted. I had seen more vultures during those weeks than I had in my entire life.

This person's skeleton, probably a man's by the size of it, was not disturbing or scary to me as it should have been. I had seen far worse than bleached bone and vacant eye sockets. No, this man's skeleton was only sad. A sad reminder of the disaster I'd survived that so many people hadn't. I grabbed a handful of candies before hurrying out of the store. The building felt like a tomb and I wouldn't go back in if I could help it.

Kiyahe watched me as I walked towards the fire and the empty chair that was waiting for me. He must've known that I had looked behind the counter anyways. But all he could've seen on my face was a look of sadness, no fear or disgust. He didn't ask me about it and I didn't bring it up. Shilah cooked a stew over the fire with smoked meat, potatoes, and carrots from the bus. After we ate, we talked about the Comanche some more and snacked on the junk food Kiyahe had brought out. Shilah was the first to go to bed, tired after having driven all day. Neka followed less than an hour later, leaving Kiyahe and I alone by the fire.

Kiyahe stared at the blazing base of the fire while I watched the sparks fly from the top and fizzle out in the lukewarm air. Fall was beginning, but the summer heat wasn't leaving without a fight. Finally, he turned and looked at me.

"Where do you want me to sleep tonight?" he asked quietly.

I turned my eyes to his and we just stared at each other for a moment. His eyes glowed warmly in the light of the fire. Like the reflection of a Tiki torch flame on Caribbean waters. He kept his face blank, showing no emotion. One side of his face glowed like melted caramel in the light of the fire while the other side was hidden in shadowed darkness. His tousled, raven black hair moved slightly in the breeze. His forehead and the high planes of his cheeks were smooth and even. Looking into his face, I could see the strong, loyal, good-hearted person that he was. But I could also see the guardedness. The caution.

After the disaster I had slept every night restlessly until I'd found the wolf. He had become my companion and protector and slept by my side every night until I found the Potawatomi. I slept much better with the wolf by my side than I had alone. And when I'd found the tribe, I had stayed with Mahala, the widowed mother of Hiawassee. Hiawassee was the brightest and sweetest little girl I'd ever met, and she had slept by my side while I stayed there. I thought of her as the little sister I'd never had. Then Kiyahe and I had gone on our "bonding journey" and I was back to sleeping on my own. I couldn't stand it, feeling alone again after all that time. It made me feel on edge, almost panicky. I had convinced him to sleep in the tent with me, and that's what we had done. Sleep and nothing more. When we'd come back I'd slept a final night with Hiawassee and now I was alone again.

But we couldn't sleep together anymore. For several reasons. One, because the twins would notice, and I didn't know whether they would say something about it, either to us or to Kiyahe's parents when we got back. Kiyahe's parents had forbidden that anything more than friendship form between us. Because we were supposed to be entirely focused on our jobs and not each other. And two, because I didn't know what sleeping with Kiyahe by my side might do to me emotionally. I didn't want to subject myself to more rejection.

"You shouldn't sleep with me," I answered truthfully, averting my eyes to the fire.

"No, I shouldn't. But I didn't ask what I *should* do, I asked what you *want* me to do to," he said, his eyes still glowing and guarded.

I sighed, "I want you to sleep where you *should* sleep. In one of the bunks."

He betrayed no emotion, only nodded and returned his gaze to the fire.

We said nothing more after that. I waited for him to go to bed first but then realized he was probably waiting on me; he wouldn't leave me alone out there unprotected. I waited a few more minutes and then excused myself to go to bed.

After I'd changed into pajamas and was curled up snugly under the covers, I waited for the sound of Kiyahe going to bed. It came just a few minutes later and I closed my eyes, willing sleep to overtake me.

In truth I was tired. Tired from the drive, tired from the stress, tired from warring what I wanted to do with what I should do.

The bed was cold, and I was alone.

I opened my eyes and stared up at the ceiling, waiting for the night to pass over.

と)

In the dream I was a child, maybe six years old at the most. I was at the lake with my grandpa who was trying unsuccessfully to teach me how to fish.

The lake was called "Rushmore Lake" and was about two miles south of the train tracks and half a mile north of Pine River. We were maybe five miles from Atlantis, South Dakota, my home town. The July air was hot and humid, the sky covered with a thick grey blanket of clouds. It trapped the heat over us and made the sweat dew up on our foreheads. The breeze picked up a bit, and every few seconds I thought I had felt a drop of rain on my arm. The storm was coming, and grandpa had told me this was the best time to go fishing. He'd explained that the rain would wash the worms and bugs from the muddy banks into the water. The fish would eat them all up like a feast.

When you are in doubt, be still and wait; when doubt no longer exists for you, then go forward with courage. So long as mists envelop you, be still; be still until the sunlight pours through and dispels the mists, as it surely will. Then act with courage.

–Ponca.

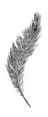

Chapter Two

I had thought that I was done having strange dreams after having found the Potawatomi and discovering my purpose.

Obviously, I was wrong.

When I woke from my restless sleep, I noticed that the bedroom was pitch black and that the only sounds were of my own breathing and the deep snores from the boys beyond my door.

I had no idea what time it was, but I knew there would be no more sleep that night for me. So I stared up at the black ceiling, waiting for dawn and thinking about my strange dream.

It was similar to the ones I'd had on my journey from South Dakota to Oklahoma in that it was both vivid and lucid. The sights, sounds, and feelings were all very sharp and I could remember them with perfect clarity after I'd awoken. And, just like the others, I had no idea how I'd conjured up such a dream or what it meant.

But unlike my other dreams, this one included a real memory. It was a perfect recollection of my grandfather, the lake, and my childish impatience. The dream had played out just like my memories of the experience, but then, for some reason, it had re-played itself with an alternate ending. One that confused, scared, and exhilarated me.

As unsettling as the storm and the battle with the fish (or rather the people) was, it had also filled me with a sort of hope. A sort of determination. The elderly Native man had said, "Be patient and calm," and his words had rung with wisdom and truth.

In the dream I had wrestled with what was on the end of the hook. And then panicked at the thought of losing the catch or being drowned in the lake. But then help had come. My protector was there, and I had realized that I wasn't alone. The feeling of those strong arms around me gave me the sense of calm that I needed to save myself and save my catch.

The old man was right.

I pondered all this while the sky gradually brightened and the boys began to toss and turn in their sleep outside my door. The accordion blinds on the windows on either side of the bedroom blocked out most of the light. But as the sun rose higher, the dim light began to brighten and permeate through the blinds and chase away the shadows in the corners. I waited to get up until the boys awoke and moved about the bus, talking in hushed whispers.

Today was the day. We were going to meet the Comanche and try to convince them of our impossible prophecy and persuade them to ally with us so that we could claim and defend this land as our own. As a nation of one people, working together to rebuild ourselves.

I pushed the strange dream out of my mind and averted my thoughts to the task ahead. I quickly dressed, mumbled my good mornings to Kiyahe and the twins, and walked through the bus and out to the gas station so that I could use the sink to brush my teeth and freshen up. The three of them had been discussing which twin should accompany us to the reservation and which one should stay behind when I passed them and walked out into the brisk morning. Kiyahe wordlessly left them to follow me and the twins continued their conversation with less than a moment's pause.

When I came out of the women's restroom, Kiyahe popped the rest of a Honey Bun into his mouth and followed me back to the bus. Our cordiality was about as warm as the icy morning air.

It was decided that Neka would accompany us to the reservation and Shilah would stay behind with the bus. With parting goodbyes and wishes for good luck, Kiyahe, Neka, and I left Shilah behind and headed down a nearby dirt road to the Comanche reservation.

"You'd better be prepared to drive that bus like a stock car and not a tractor if we come running back!" Neka shouted back over his shoulder.

Shilah rolled his eyes at his brother and Neka snickered as we walked down the road away from the bus. I swung my elbow into Neka's side, "That's not funny, Neka. Knock it off," I scolded. And my expression must have looked as nervous as I felt because his smile disappeared, and he stared at his shoes from then on as we walked.

As we made our way to the reservation, Kiyahe watching for danger and Neka watching his shoes, I tried to form a halfway competent speech in my head. Public speaking was not my forte and I didn't want to blabber like an idiot when the time came.

We made it to the outskirts of the reservation, a few people walking to and from the dilapidated houses and trailers that looked very much like the homes of my new tribe. As we neared, several people caught sight of us and stared. I guessed they would wonder who the two men were that they didn't recognize as their own. But mostly, I assumed they were staring at me. The first white woman they'd seen in almost two months.

Their stares burned straight through to my bones.

An older man, about the same age as Kiyahe's father, walked briskly towards us. His fists were balled tightly at his side and his eyes were narrowed into slits as he glared at me.

We stopped walking and let him come to us. Kiyahe moved to stand in front of me, his hands raised to the man as if to say, "We come in peace." Neka moved to my side, so close his shoulder was pressed against mine. I saw his hand twitch for the pistol in his jacket. I flexed my own hand, resisting the urge to slip the bow off of my shoulder where it hung like a sash.

"What's your business here?!" The man nearly shouted at us from where he stopped about ten feet away from Kiyahe. His piercing eyes had turned from me to Kiyahe when he spoke.

"We mean no harm. We only come to see your chief," Kiyahe answered calmly.

"What for?" the man challenged, his nostrils flaring.

"She brings a message for him," Kiyahe responded without taking his eyes off the man to gesture to me.

The man returned his steely gaze to me. I flinched and roughly cleared my throat. "I…it's true. I need to speak with your chief immediately, will you take us to him…please?" I stammered.

The man snarled under his breath before turning on his heel and walking away. Kiyahe waved his hand for us to follow, still not taking his eyes off the man. Neka had to give me a slight push to get my feet to move. His shoulder brushed mine as we walked into the reservation.

The scene was reminiscent of when I had first walked into the Potawatomi reservation nearly a week before then. The people stared at me in shock, some baffled, some angry, some murmuring to each other in rushed whispers, some running inside homes to inform others of the strange white visitor, all while an unfriendly man led me in and I blushed beet red under their scrutiny.

Last time I had stared at my feet and watched them through my peripherals. This time I tried to appear strong and unafraid. I raised my chin in an effort to look confident but not arrogant and I made eye contact with as many of the onlookers as I could. Some glared at me as I did, others looked away in embarrassment. I looked to my protectors for their reactions. I couldn't see Kiyahe's eyes, but his head was aimed straight at the grouchy man. Being the diligent protector that he was, I guessed he was watching the growing crowds through his peripherals, looking for the first sign of danger. His hand twitched spasmodically by his side, ever ready to reach for his grandfather's pistol in its concealed holster inside his jacket. Neka looked all around us in awe, this tribe was far more populous than ours and I guessed he was looking for danger as well.

Oddly enough, my fear didn't totally consume me. Perhaps it was my growing trust in my selfless protectors or perhaps it was the déjà vu of having walked through a reservation like this one before. The Potawatomi hadn't chased me away or killed me, and I had hope that the Comanche wouldn't either.

In the back of my mind, I did notice one key difference from my home tribe and this tribe. Although their numbers were easily double or triple what ours were, there were not thousands here as we'd expected. Several hundred to be sure, but not thousands. The proof of that was in the occasional charred or pulverized home that we passed as we walked through the reservation. The rickety foundations that remained were just as ghostly and dispiriting as all the other structural remains I had seen in the last month and a half. I quickly did the math in my head, counting the livable homes that we passed and estimating how many people could live in each one. Even if you put as many as ten people in the tiny homes, it didn't add up to even one thousand people.

The grouchy man stopped us in front of a double wide trailer and commanded that we wait outside while he spoke with the chief. We did as we were told, watching the crowds go back to their daily lives, one person or so at a time. Kiyahe kept his eyes glued to the trailer door while Neka watched the crowds. I fervently rehearsed my speech in my head while chewing my fingernails.

After what felt like a very long time, but was probably only five minutes or so, the grouchy man came out looking less furious but still very angry.

"The chief will speak with you, but we ask that you leave your weapons outside."

"We can't do that, I'm afraid," Kiyahe answered sternly. "We have a sworn obligation to protect this woman and are risking enough by coming here outnumbered."

The grouchy man's face flushed and his nostrils flared. He opened his mouth to make his request a demand, but a soft voice spoke from inside the open door to the trailer stopped him. He hunched his shoulders in defeat and waved us in without another word. The three of us filtered into the home, Kiyahe leading the way, Neka taking up the back.

I was instantly reminded of a nursing home when we stepped inside. The stagnant heat was too much for the small space and the air smelled of dust and soap. The interior of the living room was done in 1970's fashion; shaggy moss green carpet, paneled walls, plain particle-board end tables, brass-based lamps, and yellowed lampshades. A faded couch with orange paisley print sat vacant along one wall. A box TV sat on a wooden TV stand in the corner across from the door. Better Homes and Gardens magazines covered the end tables. The lighting was dim but homey, the room aged but purposeful. To the left, across the room from us, sat the chief and his wife in brown, threadbare rocking armchairs.

A quiet gasp escaped my lips when I looked at the chief's face. He was elderly, seventy or eighty years old. His skin a leathery brown but papery in texture. A handful of age spots and sunspots sprinkled his face. His eyes were deep-set and a bottomless black. His peppered eyebrows were thick and full. His thinning, wispy silver hair moved with even the slightest breeze or movement.

He was the same elderly Native man from my dream the night before.

"Hello," The chief said in a sandpapery voice, barely louder than a whisper. Even the sound of his voice was exactly like my dream. "I am Chief Cheveyo of the Comanche, and this is my wife." He gestured to her, but I could not tear my wide eyes away from his too familiar face to look at her.

I barely registered Kiyahe's words as he introduced us and asked that the chief listen to our story and consider our request. My mind was running sporadically, trying to figure out how I had dreamt of this man before meeting him and why.

Neka nudged me with his elbow, startling me out of my reverie. I suddenly realized that everyone was looking at me and waiting for me to speak. I gulped quite audibly and took a step forward toward the chief. Kiyahe stepped forward as well, as if tethered to me by an invisible rope.

"H...hello sir. My name is K...Kaya," I gulped again. His expression showed nothing but patience. I glanced at his wife then, who smiled at me in encouragement. She looked to be the same age as him; her skin, hair, and eyes a feminine version of her husband's. The only difference I noted between them was how they were dressed, he in traditional Native garb and her in simple, grandmotherly clothes.

I took a slow, deep breath through my nose, trying to calm my nerves and arrange my words so that I wouldn't babble like an imbecile. I had totally forgotten the semi-formed speech I had mentally prepared. When I'd taken one breath, and then a second, I heard the distant howl of a wolf.

My body froze but my head whipped back and forth between the boys, my eyes wide with surprise at a sound that I hadn't heard in so long. My lips started to form the words, "Did you hear that?" but no noise came out. Both boys looked back at me with concern, like I was crazy, obviously oblivious to the howl. The chief, his wife, and the grouchy man also conveyed ignorance of the noise. I looked towards the back window as if I could see my wolf loping through the brush just outside. He wasn't there. I wondered if I'd imagined the howl but immediately rejected the notion. I *had* heard him. And, more than that, I could *feel* him. I could feel a small bit of the strength and hope that I had felt back when he was by my side. The feeling spread all the way from my fingers through my toes.

It calmed me.

It re-focused me.

It gave me the courage to straighten my spine and square my shoulders before returning my gaze to the chief and continuing.

I stuttered my way into my story of how I'd survived the disaster, my voice dropping to a whisper when I spoke of losing my parents and starting my journey away from home. But as I continued, my voice grew stronger and I could hear the truth in my words and feel it mirrored in my eyes. They listened politely, even the grouchy man in the corner relaxed as I spoke. But when I told them of the legend and my tribe's unwavering belief in it, their expressions started to morph.

The chief's thick eyebrows knitted together in suspicion and his wife looked from me to her husband in question. The grouchy man in the corner's breathing accelerated and I could feel Kiyahe and Neka tense behind me. I kept on explaining, my plea for understanding saturating my words.

"And so you are the first tribe we have visited in our journey. We need your promise for an alliance and support for me as your leader to continue. Can you honor us with that?" I asked in conclusion.

Everyone was frozen except for Cheveyo who sucked in a deep breath as if my long spiel had tired him greatly. He looked at me scrupulously for several long moments.

"This is ridiculous!" The grouchy man suddenly shouted from his corner. Everyone jumped except for the chief. "You can't honestly believe this hogwash!" the grouchy man sneered. Everyone turned to look at the man except for Cheveyo and I who watched each other intently.

The grouchy man began insulting me, his volume growing with his anger. Kiyahe tried to interject and defend me but it only made the man more infuriated. The urge to smile came to me then, but I fought it and won. Kiyahe had acted just like this man was acting when I'd said my piece to the Potawatomi just a few weeks ago. But now he shouted in defense of me. The argument continued for a minute or two before Cheveyo raised his hand. The grouchy man and Kiyahe were instantly silenced.

"I think what is best," Cheveyo croaked in the loudest voice he could manage, "is to let the tribe vote. What you ask of us affects us all and we will need time to consider. Please, let us host a dinner for you tonight as our honored guests and you can tell your story to the tribe as a whole."

It wasn't the automatic "yes" we were hoping for, but we respected his decision. We left in peace, promising to come back that evening for the feast and to repeat our story. The grouchy man smiled slyly at me in parting but said nothing and did not follow us. It was obvious he would be promoting a "no" vote throughout the tribe for the next several hours.

There were less onlookers as we headed out of the reservation and most looked at us now with resigned curiosity. Kiyahe and Neka never let down their guard but I tried to smile at some of the Comanche in a friendly gesture. The strength and calm from the wolf continued to run through me until we left the outskirts of the reservation.

Shilah was chomping at the bit for the run-down of what had happened when we got back. Neka filled him in on every detail while Kiyahe sat in a camp chair outside, on the lookout for anyone who might have followed us or decided to come visit. I locked myself in my bedroom and watched him from one of the windows.

Ever since our "bonding journey," I had never doubted that Kiyahe would protect me. But I'd never expected the diligence and intensity of that protection. Kiyahe didn't just put himself between me and whatever threat that was posed against us, the way Neka did. He moved with me like a magnet and defended me not only physically, but verbally. When the grouchy man in the chief's trailer had started hurling insults at me, Kiyahe defended me vehemently, even thought it was not really necessary. Not once had I heard him or either of his parents say that he had to defend my reputation and protect me emotionally.

And in retrospect, his decision to do so might not have been the smartest thing to do. When he'd argued right back with the grouchy man, it had made the man grow even more agitated. If it wasn't for Cheveyo commanding their silence (impressively with nothing but raising his hand) I wondered if a fist fight would have ensued. Surely Kiyahe had noticed that arguing with the man had done nothing but increase the tension in the trailer, increasing the chance that violence might erupt.

So why had he done it? I could have easily turned on the grouchy man and defended myself, slinging my fair share of words back at him. The only reason I didn't was because his opinion was not the most important one to us in that moment. Kiyahe knew I was plenty capable of holding my own with words. Had he worried that Cheveyo might take the man's opinions into consideration?

Or maybe, just maybe, had he been verbally protective of me because he cared about me? Maybe he didn't care what the man or even the chief thought. Maybe he cared that I would take the insults to heart.

I watched Kiyahe through the window with admiration. I was reminded that Kiyahe wasn't just my protector and friend, he was a truly good person.

And he deserved more than a cold shoulder. I swore to myself then that I would try harder not to be so coarse and surly with him. Maybe we would even figure out how to be friends without crossing that feather thin line into something more.

Before we left for the reservation again, Kiyahe had the three of us dress in traditional Native wear. I wore a borrowed buckskin dress from Mahala, adorned with fringes and beading. It complemented the turquoise and aquamarine necklace she had made and given me before we'd left Oklahoma. I hadn't once taken it off since she gave it to me. Kiyahe wore buckskin pants, sewn together on the sides with leather ties. He wore no shirt (which I tried not to be distracted by) but donned a breast plate with rib bones from some animal or other, running horizontally from the hollow at his neck all the way to his waist. Neka wore soft leather pants and a cowhide poncho-shaped shirt with intricate Aztec-like patterns and fringes. All three of us wore weathered moccasins with more fringes.

Two months ago, I would have thought I looked ridiculous in these clothes. I would have felt like I was wearing a costume and not evening formal wear.

But now I felt the honor of dressing like the people. *My people.* I felt like I'd been transported back through time and was much wiser than I really was. The ancient Potawatomi shaman woman who'd predicted my arrival 200 years ago would have expected Kaya to look as I did now. Except maybe tanner, with long black hair, and midnight colored eyes.

We left Shilah with the bus again, feeling more optimistic than we had this morning. But even so, Neka kept his jokes and snide comments to himself. I left my bow behind but Kiyahe and Neka still carried their pistols.

The three of us walked into the reservation as the sun was setting. Streaks of brilliant orange and pink raced off into the horizon, the clouds nothing but feathery white wisps in the sky. The people were lighting kerosene lamps and hanging them outside their doors or setting them on their porches. They were dressed in traditional clothing like us, although some had gone even further and painted their faces in various patterns of blue, red, and gold, their tribal colors as Neka had whispered to me in explanation. Not war paint, ceremonial paint. A good sign.

We walked to the chief's trailer, unsure of where everyone was supposed to meet. He greeted us like we were old friends, shaking our hands. His wife hugged me delicately and smiled but did not speak. They escorted us to a large meeting hall in the center of the reservation, "The Lodge," as they called it. Inside there were rows upon rows of folding tables and chairs set up. Like the Potawatomi did for their ceremonies, there was a head table facing all the others. Seven chairs aligned one side of the table, an American flag stood in one corner behind the table and the Comanche flag stood in the other corner.

We took our seats, Cheveyo and I in the middle, my protectors flanking my side and Cheveyo's family flanking his. The chief said grace shortly after the last stragglers had come in the door and taken their seats. The meal was served immediately after that, Kiyahe tasting my food and drink to make sure they were safe for me.

After the meal, Cheveyo announced that all children ages fifteen and younger were to go to the adjacent room, the older children in charge of watching the younger ones. After they left, he motioned that I should stand and tell my story. I stood with shaky knees and took a deep breath. Hundreds of eyes were on me and I could feel a clammy layer of sweat on the back of my neck. I wrung my hands together behind the table where the people couldn't see them.

And then I felt the warm caress of Kiyahe's finger on the back of my left hand. It was there for less than a second, and I looked down at him in question. He gave me an encouraging nod before turning his gaze back on the people. His touch had startled me at first, like the wolf's howl had earlier. But then I felt a warm calm spread through me, also like earlier. I took a second deep breath and eased into my story. Despite the large crowd, telling it was easier this time. Perhaps practice was the key. Perhaps when we were at the end of our journey, after having told it many times over, I would be able to tell it flawlessly.

I tried to look at each individual in the crowd. All seven hundred of them, as Kiyahe had estimated. Kiyahe's father, Ahote, had been right, not all tribes had come out of the disaster unscathed. I tried to take that knowledge of their loss and relate it to my own loss, to further convince them that I was on their side. As I spoke, their faces gradually softened and I hoped, just a little bit, that they would come to empathize and agree with my words. To see the bare honesty in them. I finished my speech with the same request I had made to the chief.

Not a single person made a sound or whisper when I sat down. The chief let the silence last a few moments, then stood to address his people.

"This is a very important and life altering decision, which is why I have decided to let all adults in the tribe vote, as it affects us all. I encourage you to sleep on it and pray to the Great Spirit for guidance. Tomorrow morning, each of you may bring a slip of paper with your name and a "yes" or "no" vote as to whether you feel our tribe should support this young woman. My two sons will count the votes over the course of the afternoon, and I will announce the final tally at this time tomorrow. You are dismissed."

At once the people disbursed or fell into hushed murmurs. Kiyahe rose from his seat and Neka and I followed his lead. We bid the chief and his wife goodnight and promised to return in the morning. Surprisingly, Kiyahe and Neka were even more alert than before as they escorted me out of the Lodge. Probably because now everyone knew what my purpose was there.

We walked in silence back to the bus, Shilah once again demanding all the details of the banquet. Neka divulged everything to him while Kiyahe and I went to our rooms to change. When I came out of my room, Shilah and Kiyahe were discussing whether it was safe for us to have a fire that night. Kiyahe won the debate and we did not have a fire. The twins played cards at the booth, I curled up on Shilah's couch biting my finger nails in worry, and Kiyahe watched the windows, always on guard.

When I heard Neka yawn and saw Shilah's eyes drooping, I suggested that we all go to bed. Kiyahe and I left the twins to their couches and walked back to our rooms. Once Kiyahe closed the door between the main room and the bunk room, I turned to him and spoke softly so that the twins couldn't hear us.

"Thank you, Kiyahe."

"For what exactly?" he asked just as softly.

"For everything today. For protecting me, and sticking up for me in the trailer, and for comforting me at the banquet..." I was glad for the darkness of the room as I felt a blush spread up my throat and over my face.

"You don't have to thank me, Marie. It's my job," he said tersely.

His tone irked me, but I reminded myself that I couldn't blame him for his gruff attitude when I'd been so sour to him. I ignored the tone and responded as softly and earnestly as before. "Well I'm grateful anyways. And I'm glad you're here." But before he could get the wrong idea, I clarified. "To protect me."

He was silent then and I wondered if I'd said too much. Or maybe not enough. Ah, hell! I had no idea what I was doing!

I turned to head to my bedroom then, my face flaming, when his hand reached out and brushed mine in the dark. I froze, and he froze.

"You're welcome," he said softly.

I smiled, even though he couldn't see it. We said nothing more after that. He went to bed in the bunk room, and I in my bedroom.

I had the same dream as the night before, but this time I was ready for it. I thought I slept a little better, but I still woke with a start long before it was time to get up. Our morning routine repeated itself. And in no time at all, it was time to go back to the Comanche reservation.

Neka suggested that we do something to help the Comanche while we waited for the votes to be counted. Kiyahe agreed and, after speaking with the chief, we were put to work alongside the people. We spent the afternoon tearing down obliterated homes and buildings, patching holes that the meteors had left behind in roofs and walls, and listening to the peoples' stories of loss and survival as we went.

The strength, assiduousness, and faith of the Comanche was both baffling and admirable to me. I had felt so alone with the loss of my parents and hometown, especially after I'd found the Potawatomi and learned that everyone in their tribe had survived. Now I was working shoulder to shoulder with people who had lost just as much, if not more, than I had.

I remembered back to those first days after the disaster. How my subconscious had kept me going, kept me living, even when my heart didn't want to. Now I felt ashamed and weak for having felt that way back then, for not caring whether the flame that was my life blew out or not. These people were fighters, whose flames had only blazed brighter. I had no doubt we would meet more people like them throughout our journey.

When the sun started to dip behind the horizon and it was almost time to attend another feast and hear the results of the vote, a young couple we'd been working alongside for most of the day offered to let us use their bathroom and shower to freshen up. We were exhausted and covered in dirt and sweat from head to toe, so we accepted graciously. Every muscle in my body ached from the hard work. And before I'd thought myself in such great shape after my original journey on foot! But the ache was not entirely unpleasant. I was sore yes, I would probably feel worse tomorrow, yes, but I felt like I had really earned the respect of the people we'd helped. We could only hope now that the vote reflected that.

We hadn't had time to run back to the bus to change into traditional clothing, but at least we were clean when we walked in and took our seats from the night before. Cheveyo and his wife smiled widely at us and their expressions filled my heart with hope.

The meal was served and this time, the children were allowed to stay, and drinks were poured, mixed, and passed around. Cheveyo was not one to torture us with suspense, he gave a very short speech about what made an honorable leader, listing and complimenting me with all the adjectives that applied to a great leader. And then he thanked the Great Spirit and the open-mindedness of his tribe, announcing that the Comanche would ally with Kaya and support her as the leader of the people.

There were cheers, claps, and whoops from all around the room. The sounds of celebration filling the air. I flushed pink with happiness and relief, thanking Cheveyo and his wife profusely for their support. The party came into full swing then, tables whisked away and chairs shoved to the edges of the room. A band of teenagers in the tribe began playing live music in a corner and dancers filled the center of the room. In my happiness I flung my arms around Kiyahe, who hugged me back tightly and whispered his congratulations in my ear. I was exultant, and also very aware of Kiyahe's warm arms around my waist and the strength with which he held me. Remembering myself, and the hundreds of other sets of eyes in the room, I backed out of our embrace and hugged Neka as well. It was much less enthusiastic, but I hoped it would dispel any ideas that Kiyahe and I were an item. I wanted it to look like I was giving out hugs to everyone and not just my favorite guardian and protector.

still strongly aware of his presence. The heat of his hands, one holding mine out, the other molded around my waist, was ten times hotter than the tingling warmth of the whiskey in my stomach. As the song continued, my senses quieted my brain and I began to relax in increments. The warmth and music working their peaceful magic on me.

After a while, Kiyahe gently broke the silence with a soft-spoken comment. "You really won them over," he nearly whispered. I could hear the admiration in his voice and a small swell of pride at his approval welled up in me.

I gave in and looked up into his liquid turquoise eyes, smiling elatedly. "It wasn't as hard as I'd thought it would be. I just needed to be patient and calm and believe everything would turn out," I admitted.

We returned to our silence as the song neared its end. I closed my eyes sleepily.

That was when I felt the heat of his hand leave my waist and gently brush my cheek with the back of his fingers.

I stiffened with shock, unable to stop my reaction. My eyes flew open and I looked up at him in question. Had that really just happened? Had he really just caressed my face like that? On purpose? In front of all these people? The question in my eyes and the chaos in my head and heart were intensifying as Kiyahe leaned his face towards mine.

No! No, no, no, no. Not here! Not in front of all these people. Not now!

I jerked away from my protector in panic, suddenly intensely aware of my surroundings. Of the fact that there were still dozens of people in the room possibly watching us. I glanced around nervously, my eyes as big as a deer's in the headlights. Would these people instill their confidence and hopes for the future in an immature, love-sick teenager? I shook my head with worry; worry of what the Comanche might think, worry that I *liked* Kiyahe's touch, worry that I *wanted* more of it. I stiffly backed away from him as the song ended. He looked at me with a mixture of concern and hurt, his liquid turquoise eyes hardening into turquoise stones. I felt a stab of guilt and pain at rejecting him, but I could not deny that this was not smart. My eyes burned with tears and I furiously tried to blink them away. Before he or anyone else could see me cry, I whirled on my heel, so fast that the room spun through my intoxicated vision.

I nearly jogged from the room, out into the cool night air, and down the road in the direction of the bus. I'm sure he and Neka followed me, but I didn't dare turn around to check. I flung open the door on the bus and ignored Shilah's startled expression as I whisked past him to my bedroom. I slammed the door behind me and buried my face in a pillow before the torrent of tears, tears of worry and desire, overwhelmed me.

May the stars carry your sadness away, may hope forever wipe away your tears, and above all; may silence make you strong.

–Chief Dan George, Salish.

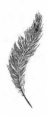

Chapter Three

I cried myself to sleep in my clothes that night, no one dared to come into my room to check on me. The next morning, I made one last trip to the Comanche reservation to say my goodbyes and final thank you's. Kiyahe and Neka followed me wordlessly there and back.

The drive to New Mexico was quiet and awkward, even more so than the drive to Texas had been. Kiyahe and I never spoke of my running away from him on the dance floor and the twins were smart enough not to ask about it or bring it up. The tension was almost palpable in the bus and the twins were unusually well behaved for the duration of the drive. There was no bickering or taunting. Come to think of it, there was almost no discussion between anyone at all. Occasionally Shilah or Kiyahe would ask Neka how much farther, as he was the one driving today, and Neka would answer. That was it. Neka kept his attention on the road, Shilah buried his face in a Sudoku puzzle book, and Kiyahe and I almost never glanced away from our windows.

Despite the endless silence, the next leg of our journey was not as long and Neka was indeed a faster driver than Shilah. We pulled into an empty RV campground a little over a mile from the Apache reservation several hours before sunset. We got out and stretched our legs, Kiyahe went for a walk to scout out the area and I helped the twins set up a campfire and chairs. When Kiyahe came back with nothing to report, I announced that I wanted to go on a walk as well.

"So, what do you think the Apache will be like?" Shilah asked, obviously trying to direct my mind to the task at hand.

"I don't know," I answered, allowing him to distract me, "It sounds like a toss up to me."

The night before, at the alliance party with the Comanche, I had asked a few men about their western neighbors and our next tribe to visit. Most had said that the Apache were known for keeping to themselves and looking out for their own. And no one had had contact with the Apache since the Fire Rains. Cheveyo had known the chief's name to be Elsu. But that was the extent of everyone's knowledge.

Cheveyo had also written, signed, and given a letter to us to show to any tribal leaders who might not be as accepting as he was. He said that it might help us along the way if we could prove the support of our allies. Kiyahe seemed to think the letter was a valuable tool to have, but I didn't share his optimism. How would any other chiefs know whether we wrote and signed the letter ourselves or whether it was real?

We made the full circle then and took our seats by the fire with Kiyahe and Neka. Shilah, still thinking about the Apache, talked strategy with Neka. Kiyahe stared into the fire, listening but not commenting. I stared at the horizon until the sun finally touched it. We ate light that night, roasting hot dogs on spits over the fire.

I excused myself to bed first, tired from all the excitement with the Comanche and from sleeping restlessly two nights in a row. I cracked the windows in the bedroom, it was a relatively warm night, and I hoped the sound of the wind in the trees would lull me to sleep.

But instead of the gentle breeze, I heard Kiyahe and the twins talking about me.

"So, what's the deal with you two being all weird when you're together? You obviously like each other. Why can't you just tell each other how you feel?" Shilah asked.

"Yeah kiss and make up already, the bickering is getting old," Neka added.

I stiffened in my bed. My efforts to look indifferent towards Kiyahe hadn't worked at all. The twins had noticed the pull between us. And they had also noticed our pathetic attempts to hide it.

"You two are wrong, Marie doesn't feel that way about me," Kiyahe said sternly, his intention to shut down the conversation clear in his tone.

But the twins were not deterred. Neka sputtered and erupted into laughter while Shilah spoke loudly over him, "Kaya might as well have it tattooed on her forehead, she's so in love with you!"

"Yeah and save us the bull and don't bother denying that you love her too!" Neka nearly shouted.

"Shut up!" Kiyahe growled at them, their laughter stopping immediately. "You two don't need to be so damn loud," he admonished.

My ears strained to hear their words after that as they spoke in hushed tones.

"Ok ok, but seriously dude, don't lie to us," Neka said, all humor gone from his voice.

"There's nothing wrong with how you feel, man, she really is a catch. Beautiful inside and out," Shilah encouraged.

I was thankful that they couldn't see me blush or see that I was awake and eavesdropping.

"It's not that simple," Kiyahe told them.

"Why isn't it?" Shilah asked.

There was a moment of silence while Kiyahe organized his thoughts.

"Because we're supposed to be focused on our jobs. If either of us loses sight of what's important, what our purposes are, it could mean the end of our whole race. There's too much at risk to let our feelings be a distraction."

"But isn't what you're doing even *more* of a distraction?" Neka countered.

"Exactly," Shilah chimed in, "Instead of wasting time and energy bickering and putting up walls between you, why don't you just go with your heart and let whatever happens happen? You have jobs to do yes, but you're still human and you still have feelings."

"And trying to ignore your feelings sounds like even more of a full-time distraction to me," Neka returned.

"You might be right," Kiyahe admitted. "We would probably work better together without all the extra drama.

But it's not just about teamwork, there's also our safety to consider."

"Isn't that what we're here for?" Neka asked, a hint of humor coming back into his voice. I could almost imagine him flexing his muscles, trying to show off and lighten the mood like he always does.

"You're here to help, yes, but it's a drop in the ocean. We'll be sorely outnumbered everywhere we go. Easy to fight, easy to kill."

The boys had no response to that.

"I already know I couldn't continue on without Marie," Kiyahe nearly whispered, his voice sounding strangled. "Protecting her is not just my purpose, it's a *need* for me now. Maybe my feelings for her make be better suited to that purpose, maybe not. I don't know."

My heart lurched at this confirmation. So Kiyahe harbored the same feelings for me that I had for him. A warmth ran through me, far beyond the reaches of my blush. My core felt like a warm blaze in a fireplace.

"What I *do* know is that the prophecy said she must live to unite the people," he continued. "If that means sacrificing my safety for hers, then that's what I must do. I'm not as necessary as she is."

Wait, what the hell?! Why would he let himself think like that?!

The warmth inside me extinguished at this. I balled the sheets in my fists, infuriated that Kiyahe would think I was worth more than him. We were *all* important to this

much too afraid to let go of the handle to wipe my eyes clear. The whipping wind dried my face for me and set my eyes to watering. But then I wasn't sure if the wind was making my eyes water or if fear was.

The driver watched me through a side mirror on the boat, his sly smile stretching from ear to ear as I struggled to maintain my balance. He veered the boat left and right, sling-shotting me across the waves. I screamed at him to stop but the shrieks blew behind me in the fury of the wind. I screamed for Kiyahe then, who's face mirrored my fear for an instant. He looked frantically between me and the driver, as if waiting for the driver to recognize my distress and stop the boat. He yelled something at the man, but the man paid no attention to him, consumed with amusement at my terror.

Less than three minutes after the ride had started, I crashed. The board wobbled underneath me for a split second before dumping me off the side, my body slamming the water. The surface slapped my face so hard that black spots flooded my vision. Aside from the spots, all I could see was water rushing in all directions. I couldn't tell which way was up, I couldn't feel my arms to let go of the handle and swim in any one direction. All I could do was scream into the depths for help. My lungs burned with the water that flooded down my windpipe.

I was drowning.

I was dying.

Where was my protector? Where was Kiyahe? These last few days of overbearing protection, and now he did nothing as I drowned? What about the tribes? What would happen to them if I perished? The crushing weight of the realization that I'd failed them was heavier than the weight of the whole lake.

"No!" my waterlogged brain suddenly screamed. "I can't die now; I have to save my people! I have to live for them! I promised! I will not give up!"

Channeling the strength in every cell of my body, I pulled against the handle, trying to right myself. The weight of the water was excruciatingly heavy, the flat knee board protesting mightily against the strain, but I heaved with everything I had left in me.

With a burst of adrenaline, I wrenched myself out of the crushing water. The boat was still pulling me hastily over the surface, but I held my balance with renewed strength. After a minute of choking on water as it siphoned out of my lungs, I regained my breath and saw the two men on board.

They were wrestling for control of the boat. The throttle was still pushed down all the way, the driver trying to keep Kiyahe away from it. The men pushed and pulled each other, struggling to keep their balance as they bounced against each other and the chairs like bumper cars. The speed and crashing of the waves didn't help either of them. As soon as one got the upper hand, the other needed only to give him a good push to knock him off balance.

Neither noticed that the boat was veering for the bank on the opposite side of the lake.

I screamed at them to stop the boat, which Kiyahe was already trying to do. The man was too consumed with stopping Kiyahe to notice where the boat was headed. I tried to pull myself closer to the boat, putting one hand in front of the other on the rope that connected the handle to the back of the boat. But the rope tore into my palms and I nearly lost my hold altogether, catching the handle just in time with bloody, slippery hands.

All I could do was hope that when we crashed, Kiyahe's life would be spared.

While the men tussled, now on the floor where I could not see them, the throttle handle pulled itself back of its own accord. The boat slowed automatically before coming to a standstill in the water.

We hadn't hit the bank. We were ok.

The men stood up then, better able to balance with the gentle rocking of the waves. My rubbery arms relaxed on the handle and I sank down slightly in the water. The man glanced between the throttle and Kiyahe and I, looking stunned and betrayed.

A crowd of Native people lined the shoreline, looking at the three of us in the water with resolve. Why they were there or what they were thinking I had no idea. All I knew was that the danger was over and we were safe.

I closed my eyes and breathed a sigh of relief.

I was especially antsy and distracted the next morning as we got ready to head to the Apache reservation. The twins must have assumed I was only nervous about meeting the next tribe. But Kiyahe knew better.

"Are you ok?" he asked me quietly as I picked at my breakfast across the booth from him, pieces of muffin falling back onto a paper plate in front of me. Looking at him, I was reminded of the conversation he'd had with the twins the night before. The admission of his feelings for me. As much as I wanted to decipher and address that issue, my dream and meeting the next tribe was far more pressing and worrisome. The twins were in the bunk room getting dressed. I had heard the concern in Kiyahe's voice, but I shook my head dismissively.

"It's nothing, I just didn't sleep well last night," I told him. It wasn't completely a lie; I *wasn't* sleeping well. A small part of me wanted to tell him about my dreams but I buried the urge. The dreams made no sense and I was embarrassed to admit that Kiyahe was a part of them. And he didn't need to worry about something he couldn't fix. He needed to be focused on our task.

Either my answer or my face made it clear that wasn't all that was bothering me. Kiyahe's brilliant blue eyes burned into mine in question and I looked out the window to avoid his gaze. The twins came out of the bunk room then, continuing some conversation about how girls back home looked compared to girls out here. I casually slid out of the booth across from Kiyahe and jumped into the twins' conversation, scolding them in a motherly way for talking about girls that way.

Everyone was in agreement that Shilah should go with us to visit the Apache while Neka stayed with the bus. When we were armed and ready, we walked wordlessly to the reservation, Kiyahe and Shilah on alert the entire way.

We slowed as we reached the outskirts and I half expected someone to intercept us like the grouchy man from the Comanche had. But the few people who milled around within our view made no move to approach us. They eyed us suspiciously, their faces carved with disdain. I did my best to look friendly and peaceable, meeting their gazes with small smiles.

When we were no more than ten feet from the nearest house, a woman turned on the sidewalk and retreated into her house, the door slamming behind her, the sound of a dead bolt locking, unmistakable. Several other men and women did the same as we neared them, people hurrying away from us and double checking their locks once they were safely inside. Two mothers interrupted their daughters who were playing with each other and a handful of dolls in a front yard. The mothers swooped them up and took them inside, abandoning the dolls in the grass.

The people didn't stop watching us though. They conspicuously parted blinds or held back curtains on their windows so they could continue watching the three strangers who did not belong.

The reservation was about the same size as the last one and just as dilapidated too. I was growing used to the scenery of the post-disaster reservations, the poor living conditions becoming a normality and expectation for me now. But I never would get used to the way people stared at me as if I were an alien. A dangerous and unwelcome alien.

A thin young man, maybe two years younger than me at most, hesitated as we approached him. His bottomless black eyes showed distrust and hostility, but his half-turned torso and shaking hands showed fear. Before he could turn to run from us, Kiyahe addressed him.

"Hello sir, my name is Kiyahe and these are my friends Shilah and Kaya," he said cordially as he gestured to Shilah and I in turn. "We come in peace to speak with your chief, would you mind taking us to him?"

The young man's eyebrows knitted together in hesitation and his right foot turned halfway as if to run from us. He was obviously regretting having stuck around long enough to be addressed. The silence stretched on awkwardly as we waited for him to give us an answer.

"We truly mean no harm," I said in my sweetest voice as I stepped towards him. "If it would make you feel better you could take us to your chief's house and be on your way, we don't have to mention who directed us there," I smiled encouragingly.

When the man, who was really no more than a boy, turned his eyes to me when I spoke, his fears seemed to evaporate. He even appeared to blush as he turned to fully face me, a shy smile on his lips. "Oh no! It's not a problem, ma'am, I'll take you to him if you'd like. Follow me." His words rushed together like he was struggling to make his mouth communicate what his brain wanted to say. He offered his bony arm to me, shakily, with the same shy smile, like a thirteen-year-old with a school boy crush.

I smiled back tentatively and took his arm. I heard the air whistle through Kiyahe's teeth and felt his urgent hand grip my other arm, the one that wasn't looped through the young man's. I jerked my elbow out of Kiyahe's grasp and threw him a warning look before he could protest. He didn't reach for me again, but he moved so that he was walking only inches behind mine and the boy's interlocking arms. Probably so that he could separate me from this stranger in a second if he needed to. Which I was sure he wouldn't need to. The scrawny boy was harmless and was no match for either of my protectors. I probably could've done a fair job protecting myself if I'd had to, as lanky as the boy was. Shilah took up my left side and the four of us walked through the reservation.

The chief's small and modest house was on the far side of the reservation, so we were forced to walk almost completely through the community to reach it. The suspicion of the Apache people did not let up and neither did Kiyahe or Shilah's guard. When we finally did reach the chief's home, a house with chipped baby blue siding and yellow painted shutters, the young man gulped as he dropped my arm, the color draining from his face. The realization hit me then that he was less nervous about us as he was about his chief. The regret and anxiety that was plain on his face did not help my limited confidence.

"I'll…uhm…go and see if he's home," the boy stammered uncertainly. We waited on the sidewalk as the young man skittered up the walk to the front door, knocking on it with a shaky fist. A middle-aged woman came to the door and they spoke quietly. I could not hear what they were saying but I could see the surprise and suspicion twist the woman's features. Her eyes were unreadable, a solid color of milky blue clouding them so that the irises and pupils were hidden. I realized that she must be blind.

The woman shut the door then and the boy walked back over to us. "She said Elsu's in the backyard tending to the garden, I'll take you to him." He led the way to the back yard, this time without offering his arm to me. Kiyahe and Shilah followed at my flanks.

Wisdom and peace come when you start living the life The Creator intended for you.

—Geronimo, Apache.

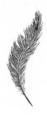

Chapter Four

Elsu was kneeling in the dirt, yanking weeds out of his small garden. He heard our approach before we reached him and rose to meet us, wiping his muddy hands on his jeans. When his eyes touched on us, his shoulders squared, and his chin rose with superiority. The corners of his mouth drooped downwards, and his eyes revealed his displeasure. I faltered in my friendly composure, shock penetrating my features. Elsu was the man from my dream the night before. The one who had driven the boat, dragging me through the lake. The one who had tried to drown me. I managed to plaster something like a smile back on my face as my thoughts ran wild.

Aside from the shock and fear that Elsu's familiarity had ignited in me, a small part of me realized that a pattern was forming between my dreams and reality. When I had been on my journey, I had seen the places I would go and the people I would meet before I got there. After hearing the legend of Kaya, I had shrugged off the peculiarity, excusing those dreams as part of the prophecy. But now I had dreamt of two different chiefs just before meeting them. The Cheveyo I met in reality was just like the Cheveyo I met in my dream. And, unfortunately, I guessed the same would go for Elsu.

"Chief Elsu, these visitors are here to see you," the young man said with a voice just barely above a whisper. He fidgeted with the sleeve of his plaid shirt. Elsu jerked his chin once and the boy pivoted and powerwalked out of the back yard, barely taking the time to throw me a yearning look as he abandoned us.

Kiyahe introduced us and explained that we brought a message and had a request for Elsu and the Apache people. When he finished, Elsu said nothing and made no motion to greet us or to give us consent to say our piece. He only stood there with his arms crossed over his barrel-shaped chest, his eyes flitting between the three of us.

When the tension became uncomfortable and the silence unbearable, Kiyahe turned and nodded to me, a sign that I should tell the chief what our purpose was.

I squared my shoulders and lifted my chin, trying to look like I knew what I was doing and that I wasn't afraid of the imposing chief. But then I worried that I might come off as arrogant, so I lowered my chin a bit and uncrossed my arms, letting them fall to my sides. I was mindful not to fidget with my jacket sleeves.

And then I heard the faintest sound of a wolf howling in the wind.

A small smile formed on my face but this time I fought the urge to look around for my former protector. I didn't look to Kiyahe or Shilah for confirmation of the sound. I knew I was the only one who'd heard it. The only one who *needed* to hear it.

Elsu's expression did not change in the slightest as I told my tale and explained the legend and our purpose for being there. When I was finished, the silence stretched out again as we held our breath, waiting for his response.

And then the chief did something none of us were expecting.

He walked away.

Without a single word.

We stood there and watched as he strolled past us to the back door of his house and went inside. The three of us stood stupidly in the chief's backyard. Shilah and I's mouths dropped open in astonishment and Kiyahe's eyebrows knitted together in confusion.

"What now?" Shilah asked. "Should we go knock on the door? Do you think he's coming back?"

No one answered him. We stood there for several minutes, watching the door the chief had walked through. Finally, Kiyahe spoke.

"I don't think he's coming back. I suppose we should leave and try again tomorrow."

We shuffled back across the back yard, watching the door as we walked, hoping the chief would come back out and stop us. Kiyahe took the lead now and Shilah and I dawdled behind him like perplexed ducklings. The boy who had taken us to Elsu's home caught up with us when we were two blocks away from the chief's house.

"So, what happened? Are you guys leaving now?" he asked dejectedly. Our disappointment must have been obvious on our faces.

We kept walking with the boy at our heels. Kiyahe acted as if the guy wasn't there. Shilah opened his mouth to answer before snapping it shut again, unsure of whether we would care if he told this boy the purpose of our visit. I decided no harm could come of answering him.

"We came to speak to your chief and ask a favor of him, but he ignored us and walked away. We might come back tomorrow to try again," I summarized. And then I had a thought, "Is there anything we could try to get through to your chief? To make him listen?" It was a long shot, but this young man had grown up in the tribe and Elsu was probably the only chief he had known in his lifetime. Maybe he could help us.

"Well Chief Elsu isn't a big talker. He's more of a man of action, you know? And he's pretty old fashioned so he puts a lot of stock into manners and all that."

Kiyahe snorted, "So what? We come back and say *please* next time?"

I threw a look at Kiyahe, he didn't need to be so cynical. But Kiyahe was ignoring me and watching the boy and the few Apache outside, scanning for danger as usual.

I had another idea then and stopped in my tracks. The young man nearly ran into me in his eagerness and Kiyahe and Shilah went less than two steps before whirling back to me.

"What if we learned some of the customs of your tribe and helped out around the reservation. Would Elsu listen to us then?" I asked the boy. Kiyahe bristled at my side but I ignored him, looking only at the lanky teenager who was our best hope for getting through to Elsu at that point.

The boy brightened at the idea, "Yes, it might help, maybe if you help the Apache, Elsu will help you. You win over the people and you might win over the chief too. It can't hurt any, I don't think."

The young man's enthusiasm was contagious, and I smiled back at him brightly. At least now we had something to work on. Shilah clapped his hands together then, also in agreeance with the idea.

"Alright then, where do we start, kid?"

⫸

For the next week we helped the Apache repair their homes and do other various projects. At first, they were leery of us and we were scarcely less leery of them. They only spoke to us when necessary and ignored my attempts to get to know them.

But Lokni, the young man who had brought us to the chief and become our tour guide of sorts, had a contagious charisma that eased the tension some when he was around. One night Kiyahe told us that Lokni's name meant "leaky roof" and that his head was most definitely leaky. The twins had rolled with laughter at that. I tried to give Kiyahe a look of disapproval, but it was hard when I was fighting a smile. Lokni wasn't the sharpest tool in the shed but he was sweet and friendly.

A couple days later, we were helping several of the men build a well when Lokni knocked an entire bag of tools off the ledge and into the well. He was immediately nominated to be lowered into the hole to retrieve the tools and Kiyahe and the men got a kick out of his obvious fear of being lowered into the dark depths by a harness made of old rope. Kiyahe suggested we leave him down there for a while and the men guffawed in agreement. I threw an elbow into his ribs for that one and made him pull Lokni up himself.

When we weren't helping the tribe repair or rebuild structures, we were taking lessons from Lokni and a few of the more outgoing men and women on Apache traditions and customs. Word was spreading of our efforts and humility and more and more of the people engaged in teaching us their ways and stepping outside their comfort zones to meet us.

At the beginning and end of each day, we went with Lokni to Elsu's home and asked to speak with him. At first his wife politely refused us each time until eventually she stopped answering the door altogether.

I felt like I had in my dream where I had almost drowned in the lake: hopeless. The dream repeated night after night and although I never actually drowned, I felt that I was. I was doing everything I could not to drown, not to fail in winning over the Apache. But none of it was getting through to Elsu.

One evening we sat around the campfire outside the bus, exhausted from the day's work. We had helped till gardens, mostly by hand as there were only a few people in the tribe with hoes or tillers. Not only was I spent physically, but mentally as well. I was getting maybe four hours of sleep a night at the most because of the recurring nightmare. It seemed now that I was familiar with the dream of drowning, my mind replayed it faster, knowing well what would happen next. Like a re-run movie. It was a relief when the dream was over, but a torture when I had no choice but to lay in the dark until it was time to get to work again.

That night Kiyahe hinted at giving up on the Apache, going on and on about how hopeless our efforts were if we couldn't get Elsu to open his door to speak with us and see how hard we were trying. He wouldn't come right out and suggest it, but I could see the gears turning in his head. It was silent when he finished venting and the twins looked to me across the fire. I simply told them we were not giving up and that we should go to bed, we weren't done there yet.

But I had to admit to myself that Kiyahe was right. Not about giving up, but about needing Elsu to *see* what we were doing and hear us out.

Ahote had given us a three-month deadline to meet all the tribes and get back to Oklahoma. If we weren't back by then, he would send people out to find us and bring us home before the thick of winter set in. We would have to return in the spring if we couldn't find and ally with all the tribes we needed to ally with.

We wanted to get this done in one trip. No one wanted to wait out the winter months wondering whether we could call ourselves united or not. The more time it took us to form a nation, the less likely the tribes would be willing to unite as one instead of reverting back to the old ways of fighting amongst each other for land. We needed to band together if we wanted any hope of reclaiming what had once belonged to the people.

I decided on a new course of action then. The next day, when we got to the Apache reservation, I asked Lokni to spread word to everyone he could and tell them to gather in front of Elsu's house. I had something to say to them. He ran off like a retriever and before long, the potholed street in front of Elsu's home was filled with people. They stretched clear down the road, the one's farthest away straining on their toes to see and cupping their ears to hear. Several fathers put their kids on their shoulders so they could see. They filled the sidewalk and Elsu's front yard, too. Neither Elsu nor his wife came out of the house. I didn't even turn to see if they were watching through the windows.

In as loud and clear of a voice as I could manage, I told the Apache the story of my survival and of the legend. I asked them the favor I had asked of their chief: to support me and to ally with me, the Potawatomi, and the Comanche in becoming one people. I explained to them why our united front was important and how important it was to me that I have their trust and be able to trust in them. As I spoke, I wondered if Elsu and his wife could hear me through the paper-thin walls of the house. I fervently hoped they could.

When I finished, the Apache people descended into conversations. As they debated amongst themselves, I saw dozens of eyes glance up at me or at Elsu's house. My plan was to ask them to try and convince their chief on my behalf. If he wouldn't speak to me, fine. But he would have a hard time ignoring seven hundred people outside his door. I would come back tomorrow. Maybe then, Elsu would have something to say to me.

But before I could make my announcement, the front door to Elsu's house swung open behind me. Swung is probably the wrong word, though. It *flew* open, the rusty hinges screaming in protest, and *whacked* into the wall behind it. I flinched, not because the sound surprised me, but because I feared the anger of the man who'd flung the door open. I didn't have to turn around to know it was the chief. Kiyahe and Shilah moved to my side, their hands twitching for their pistols. Their demeanors were proof enough.

While the sound of Elsu's slow, heavy footsteps approached behind me, I hardened my face into a determined mask. I would not let him see any fear. I had proven myself to the Apache and it wasn't my fault he hadn't been around to see it.

"I do not remember calling a tribal meeting," he hissed at my back. His voice wasn't what I'd expected. I had been prepared for a booming shout that shook my bones with its fury. Elsu didn't yell, in fact he had spoken so quietly I doubted whether anyone besides Kiyahe, Shilah, and I had heard him. He spoke in a low, menacing tone. The kind that gave you chills up and down your spine. The calm before the storm.

"In fact," he continued, "If I *had* called a tribal meeting it wouldn't have included the entire tribe. Just the elders. The elder *men*. The elder *Native* men."

I turned to look at him then. His face mirrored his anger and his stance was strong and confident. His arms were folded across his chest, the veins standing out in his russet colored forearms. His fists were clenched, the knuckles almost as white as my own skin. I wondered for a second if he would dare to hit me. Surely he wouldn't hit a woman. I hoped. And then I remembered Kiyahe at my side and I let my own posture relax. Kiyahe could surely take this man in a fight if he had to. But then I tensed up again, remembering my dream and the men wrestling on the boat. Maybe the fight wouldn't be as even as I hoped.

The nearest men in the crowd had noticed the face-off between the chief and the three of us then and a fresh wave of whispers spread through the crowd. Everyone grew quiet in their curiosity.

I wanted to shout at Elsu that I was doing what was necessary because I had a job to get done! I also wanted to tell him that he was making it a hundred times more difficult than it needed to be. If his answer was "no" then just say it to my face!

But I didn't raise my voice to him and I didn't give excuses for stepping out of line. Instead I simply said, "I'm sorry," and waited for his response.

He chewed it over for a minute and I watched every twitch in his face and glint in his eye, trying to decipher what he was thinking.

In a clear, but much louder voice, loud enough for the first several rows of people to hear he said, "I will not ally with you. You are no chief of mine." And then he turned on his heel and stalked back into the house.

He might as well have stabbed me with a knife, it would have been just as painful. Everything I had tried, and he refused to see it! The voices in the crowd spread the chief's words back and back through the rows. I heard it over and over and each time it was like the knife was twisting.

"We could call for a vote," Shilah suggested in a meek voice from behind me.

"No," I said as I shook my head and turned to him. "I will not make them choose between me and their chief. We're done here."

I stalked off into the crowd then, looking at no one and nothing but my feet. The people parted like a sea and grew quiet as I passed. I didn't look up until I was back at the bus.

Neka caught one look of my face and glanced away awkwardly. I would let Shilah fill him in, the chief's words had drained me. The simple answer to all our time here could be summed up in two words and I couldn't even utter those.

We failed.

It was several hours before anyone spoke on the bus. Kiyahe was the one to break the silence. "So, I think tomorrow we should leave for the next tribe. Maybe by the time we get back home Elsu will have changed his mind. We can come back and try again later."

No one answered. None of us truly believed Elsu would ever change his mind. We could try, of course we would try. But it looked as if this trip would never end.

I didn't agree or disagree with Kiyahe, I just took a deep breath and resolved to pull myself together before the next tribe. I went to bed early that night. It didn't take long for everyone else to follow suit.

જી

I had the same dream again as usual. It woke me up when it was still dark, so I patiently laid in bed and waited for daylight to come.

And then a pounding on the bus startled me. It woke the boys and within seconds we were flipping on lights and throwing open doors between rooms. Neka darted to the front of the bus, his hands fumbling while trying to find the right key to start the bus in case we had to floor it out of there. Kiyahe's hands were the opposite, quick and assured as he pulled three pistols out of a compartment, tossing two loaded ones to Shilah and I while he loaded a third for himself. Shilah and I fell onto a couch by the window, peering through the blinds to see who was knocking on the door. Before I could make out the shape in the dark, Kiyahe grabbed a handful of my sleep shirt and yanked me back, away from the window. "Don't let them see you!" he whispered harshly.

"It's a woman!" Shilah announced.

"How many?" Kiyahe asked, his voice all business as he thrust the clip into the gun and flipped the safety off.

"Just one from what I can see."

Kiyahe ran around to all the other windows, scanning them for other people. When he was satisfied the woman was alone, he ordered Shilah and I into the bedroom and Neka to be ready to start the bus. He answered the door as Shilah pulled me by the elbow back to my room. He didn't shut the door though; his curiosity was just as strong as mine. Who was this woman and how had she found us? What did she want? We peered through the crack and held our breath so we could hear the whispering. It did no good though, she spoke in a language neither Shilah or I understood. We kept watching eagerly, regardless.

Kiyahe spoke to her in the same strange language for just a few minutes and then he shut the door and she was gone. We stumbled out of the bedroom and Neka joined us on the couches, I was the only one to put my gun down on the dining table.

"She's Elsu's niece and she says the people threw a fit outside Elsu's house after we left. They believe our story and want to ally with us and the other tribes."

"And what did Elsu say?" I asked, fearful of the answer.

"He didn't say anything, he didn't come back outside after talking to you, even to address the shouting outside. She said the elders and most of the tribe is in agreement about having a vote. She's confident we'll win the majority."

"And?" I asked fearfully, it sounded too good to be true.

"And she wants us to come back in the morning to hear the vote. She thinks that maybe her uncle will change his mind when he has proof that most of his tribe supports you."

"I don't mean to be a Debbie Downer here, but what if it's a trap?" Neka asked.

"I'm wondering that too. It might not be safe to go back," Kiyahe agreed.

"It's not safe to go anywhere!" I shouted. What the hell were they thinking? We couldn't pass up an opportunity like this! "I could be attacked or shot at any day of the week! If they wanted to kill me, they would have done it by now."

"They didn't know why you were here until now," Kiyahe countered.

"Well now they do and now they know where we're making camp too," Shilah added.

"We should probably move the bus," Kiyahe said.

"I've got an idea," I said pointedly. "How about we go out on a limb and trust them? Just like we did with the Comanche and like we'll have to do with every other tribe we meet. If someone comes out here to attack us, we'll leave. But if they don't then I'm going back to the reservation in the morning."

"I'm not going to gamble our lives and leave the bus here to prove a point, Marie!" Kiyahe shouted.

"Fine! Move the damn bus and I'll go back to the reservation right now!" I shouted back. Kiyahe was standing in the middle of the floor over me. Just then I realized that I was straining against Shilah's grip on my elbow. I pried his fingers off so I could stand toe-to-toe with Kiyahe.

"You're making this so much harder for me than it needs to be!" Kiyahe threw his hands in the air in frustration.

"And you're doing the same to me! We have a chance to make them our allies and you're throwing it away because you're afraid! You can't keep me away from every tribe just because they don't kiss my hand and invite me in for tea the minute we meet!"

"You're so irresponsible with your life it's insane! And you're some kind of stupid if you think I'm going to let you go down there right now!"

"Well I'm not asking for your permission!" I spat. I whirled towards the door of the bus. I didn't think about the fact that it was still dark outside, or that I was in my pajamas, and especially not about what could happen to me. All I wanted in that moment was to get away from Kiyahe.

Before I could make it two steps though, strong hands grabbed my upper arms and yanked me backwards, away from the door. Kiyahe grabbed me in a bear hug and pinned me to his chest, his hands creating handcuffs around my wrists. Even the twins had gotten off the couch, ready to run after me if Kiyahe hadn't grabbed me first. I strained away from him and tried to twist my hands free, but his grip was unbreakable.

"Let me go, damn it!"

"No!"

"What the hell is your problem?!"

"I'm not losing you!" he shouted.

The twins and I froze in shock. He said it like it was a fact. A fact that tortured him. His turquoise eyes seemed darker as they begged mine to understand.

Looking into those eyes, I drooped in his arms in surrender and confusion. I understood the words. I understood the feelings behind them. But those were *my* words and *my* feelings. *I* was the one who couldn't lose *him*.

Before I could even begin to put a coherent thought together, let alone coherent words, Shilah suggested a compromise.

"How about we move the bus for the rest of the night and Kaya goes back tomorrow with me and you, Kiyahe?"

Kiyahe didn't release my eyes as he nodded his agreeance with Shilah's suggestion. When the boys retreated to the front of the bus to get it started and moved, Kiyahe finally released my wrists and turned away. I reached out to the arm of the couch to steady myself so I wouldn't slump to the floor. He went into the bunk room and ever so softly, shut the door behind him. I stood there motionless, staring at the door he'd closed behind him. After a while I realized that I wanted to go back to my room to think privately. But I was too chicken to look or speak to Kiyahe for the rest of that night. I laid on Shilah's couch and waited as they moved the bus. I must have fallen asleep again because when I woke up it was daylight. Shilah must have left me his couch and slept the remainder of the night in the bunk room.

I was the first one awake and I couldn't keep my thoughts focused on what the Apache's plans were. All I could think about was what Kiyahe had said about not being able to lose me.

I realized then that this was why we couldn't fall in love. He was willing to risk our success with the Apache because it was a risk for my safety. It was getting harder for him to accept that I was always in danger. That I was always vulnerable.

But that's how it was and how it would always be. There was nothing he could do about it and his frustration over it was breaking through that responsible, composed surface.

And he was right. I was making it harder on him. I was a monster for being so careless with my life, and in turn his feelings, last night. If the one thing he truly wanted was to keep me safe, as impossible as that was, then I should be more mindful of that. I wouldn't shy away from negotiating with the tribes. The fate of an entire race depended on me for that. But I would take Kiyahe's thoughts into consideration more.

We got ready silently that morning and no one talked about last night's argument. Kiyahe stuck to the compromise, leaving with me and Shilah to hear what the Apache had to say. He led us wordlessly along the new, longer route to the Apache reservation. And we walked into nothing short of a spectacle.

Everyone was gathered outside Elsu's house again and I could hear men shouting from up by the front door. Kiyahe led us around the edge of the large crowd up to the front of Elsu's house where several men were gathered and arguing in a language I didn't know. One by one they each turned to see us approach, Elsu in the middle, his eyes blazing at me. I flinched under the heat of his gaze.

Kiyahe spoke to them in their language and translated for Shilah and me. "Elsu has agreed to a vote but he doesn't trust anyone to count it," he explained.

Elsu's face flamed with rage and he turned on Kiyahe, "I will speak for myself, boy!" he spat.

"Then speak in a language we can all understand, *Great Chief.*" Kiyahe threw back.

That was all it took. The chief lunged at Kiyahe, his hands going for his throat. He was fast for his age, and before anyone knew what was happening, he'd knocked Kiyahe to the floor. He pinned him down under his weight and dug his fingers into Kiyahe's throat.

As strong as he was, he was outnumbered and almost as quickly as it started, the elders had pulled Elsu off of Kiyahe and Shilah and I stepped in between them. Kiyahe gasped and sputtered before grabbing my sleeve and pulling me back behind him. As much as I wanted to lunge for Elsu myself, I let Kiyahe pull me back.

"No more!" the oldest elder shouted. "I say we vote and the vote gets re-counted by each elder."

"You say nothing! You are not chief!" Elsu shouted at the old man.

"I have an idea," Kiyahe said, trying to keep the rasp out of his voice. Elsu turned his narrowed eyes on him but did not say anything or lunge at him again. "You stand on one side of the street and Kaya stands on the other. Anyone who sides with her stands behind her and anyone who doesn't stands behind you. Everyone can see the vote with their own eyes."

"No," I said then, "I will not make them choose between me and their chief. We need to be united." I looked at Elsu then. "I'm not trying to take anything away from you, Elsu. This will still be your tribe and you will still be their chief. I just want you to believe in me and be my ally, not my enemy."

"We lost *everything* to white's and their lies," he growled.

"I know, but I have no interest in taking away anything from you. I lost everything that I had, and I know *exactly* how it feels to lose everything." Tears pricked my eyes and I blinked furiously to hold them back. "I wouldn't wish that feeling on anyone else. *Especially* the Native people. Your people have given me more than I could have ever asked for and I'm doing everything I know how to pay that back. Please Elsu, I ask you to be our ally, nothing more and nothing less. I can't ask that of anyone else until I have that from you."

Everyone stood in silence for a good while after that. Elsu looked around him and I could see the relinquishment in his eyes. This was not a fight he would win, and he knew that. And after what seemed like ages, the Apache chief nodded. "I will give you our alliance and nothing more and nothing less," he said quietly. My relief and happiness lit up my face like a kid on Christmas morning. I wanted to throw my arms around him in ecstasy but I stopped myself. We were allies, he'd admitted that, but we were not friends. Not yet anyway. I extended my hand and he shook it once. He turned and made the announcement to the tribe, who whooped and hollered in agreement. Had it come to a vote it sounded as if I would have had the majority.

Kiyahe asked Elsu if he might write and sign a letter to any other chiefs we might encounter, vouching that we were trustworthy and claiming us as allies. It was a short, blunt letter but it said what we needed it to say. The chief and the elders bid us polite goodbyes and we made a final round through the crowd before we left. A tearful Lokni was the last to wish us good luck on our journey and I thanked him for all his help. Kiyahe even shook his hand before we left.

We embarked for Northern New Mexico then, the Navajo would be our next tribe to visit.

In this time, it isn't Indians versus Cowboys. No. This time it is all the beautiful races of humanity together on the same side and we are fighting to replace our fear with love. This time, bullets, arrows, and cannon balls won't save us. The only weapons that are useful in this battle are the weapons of truth, faith, and compassion.

—Lyla June, Dine', Navajo.

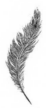

Chapter Five

The first problem we encountered with the Navajo was finding them.

While Shilah drove the bus, Kiyahe directed him according to where his father had said the reservation would be on the map. The Navajo reservation was out in the boon docks, several miles from any nearby towns, campgrounds, or gas stations. When we were, according to the map, less than a mile away, we stopped the bus alongside the road. We were out in the open, exposed, an easy target. But there was nowhere better to make camp and Kiyahe wouldn't risk us getting any closer to the reservation just yet.

The twins and I set up camp alongside the road within a small cluster of desert willow trees. The yellowed leaves provided just a small patch of shade but with fall in full swing, it wasn't the shade we really needed. It was camouflage. If curious eyes found the bus before we found the tribe, we would have to decide whether to engage them or make a run for it. Everywhere we'd camped thus far was well hidden, but here we stood out like a sore thumb in the northern New Mexican desert.

While we set up camp, Kiyahe walked a wide perimeter around us, scouting for anyone who might be near. He went out so far that I lost sight of him in the setting sun. When he came back, he looked edgy. I didn't have to ask him what was wrong, he told us as soon as he was in ear shot.

"Put the stuff back on the bus, we're leaving," he commanded. "I walked clear to the outskirts of the reservation and there's no one there. The Navajo have left."

"But why?" I asked.

Kiyahe sighed, "My father said that some tribes might not stay on their reservations now that there's more than enough room to spread out and start over. They must have left for somewhere better."

"Can't say I blame them," Neka said. "This place is a dump."

I had to agree with Neka, there was little out here to entice anyone to want to stick around. The desert land stretched from horizon to horizon with only sporadic crags and cliffs to punctuate the view. The brush and cactuses were spiny and dried up. And the constant wind, with little to break it, whipped the dust up and spun it in miniature tornadoes, coating everything. I supposed, to someone, the area was beautiful and vast. To me, in what was left of the world, it was lonely and desolate.

"We'll load up and go find them. They probably didn't go far, this is still their land after all," Kiyahe decided.

And so we loaded up and drove along the open roads and through the decimated towns, looking for the Navajo. Kiyahe had said that the tribe was nomadic back in the day and he worried, the longer that we drove, that they might not stop in a single place for long, but rather keep travelling and keep moving. It didn't help that we were confined to the roads the bus could travel.

We drove well into the night, everyone looking out the windows for any sign of the tribe. At first, as night settled in, it was hard to make out shapes in the dark. But then as the moon rose higher, its light shone unobstructed. Even with the tallest cliffs trying to block it out, its illumination cast a glow on everything beneath it. We had a few false alarms; Shilah saw a grove of small trees that looked like a band of people in the shadows, Neka saw what he thought was smoke and believed it might be coming from campfires, but the smoke was only mist that rose off of a small pond whose water was warmer than the air above it, causing a blanket of mist that hung above its surface. I almost called out myself, seeing a herd of palominos that, for a split second, appeared to have riders. But as they galloped away, their manes flying and tails swishing, I saw that they were bare-backed and rider-less. We were looking so hard for the tribe that we saw more and more false mirages.

My eyes began to droop and my forehead pressed against the glass of the window I'd been looking out of. I had no idea what time of night, or maybe early morning, it was. Just as I was about to throw in my towel and go to bed, Kiyahe pointed out the windshield from the passenger seat in the front of the bus and shouted.

"There! You see it? Campfires!"

Everyone shook off their drowsiness and crowded in front of the bus to see. The fires were small, but they were there, dwindling as they were no longer being tended to. The tribe had gone to bed in the surrounding tipis, leaving the embers and coals to burn themselves out. Faint trails of smoke wafted into the air above them.

"Park over there so that those trees are between us and them," Kiyahe directed Shilah. "Hopefully no one will walk this far out and find us, we need to get some sleep and approach them in the daytime."

"What if they take off again before we wake up?" Neka asked.

"Then we follow them again, at least we'll be a lot closer this time, though."

Everyone went to bed, but no one slept deeply, we were too anxious being this close to our next tribe. The area had more cover than the first place we'd parked but we weren't well hidden by any means.

I had another strange dream that night, and it left me with a feeling in the pit of my stomach that the Navajo weren't going to like us. And not just because we were following them.

I woke just before dawn and got myself ready to go meet our next tribe. Kiyahe was already awake, he'd found a pair of binoculars and was watching the tribe through a part in the blinds by his chair. He was dressed and ready to go, his foot tapped steadily on the floor. The twins were still asleep on their couches, but they didn't snore, and they rustled in their sleep. They would be awake soon.

"What do you see?" I asked Kiyahe quietly, coming to stand behind him and looking over his shoulder out the window. I tried to ignore the electric buzz I felt in being so close to him, focusing instead on finding the Navajo outside the window. I could see a few figures moving around and the fires burning brighter than they had the night before. But they were too far away for me to see much else.

"I think I know which one is the chief, he wears a traditional headdress," Kiyahe told me. I remembered back to the chiefs we'd met thus far, neither Cheveyo or Elsu had been wearing headdresses when we'd met them. But Kiyahe's father, Ahote wore his all the time. Perhaps some chiefs preferred to wear one all the time and others only on special occasions? "He's about the same age as my father and Elsu from what I can see." I wondered if this chief would be more understanding like Kiyahe's father or if he would be more stubborn like Elsu. I swallowed at the thought of the latter.

Kiyahe described the tribe to me as I ate my breakfast at the booth. The tribe was smaller than the Comanche and the Apache, but still larger than our own tribe. About half of the people slept in tipis, the other half in modern camping tents. When the sun had just barely left the edge of the horizon, the Navajo began packing up their camp and I woke the twins and told them to hurry and get ready. Neka would be coming with us this time, the twins had settled into a pattern of taking turns with the tribes. Kiyahe didn't like the pattern, he wanted Shilah to go with us to the larger, less friendly tribes but the twins had convinced him that Shilah's size really didn't give us a better chance of winning a fight if it came to that. We were sorely outnumbered everywhere we went and bullets don't care how big their targets are.

We waited until they began walking. After they were on the move, we left Shilah with the bus and quietly powerwalked after them.

A woman from the back happened to turn around and catch sight of us after almost half a mile. She called out and the whole tribe stopped and turned to see us. We slowed our walk and approached with our hands out in peace. The woman, strong and fearless and dressed in rugged hiking clothes, walked to meet us halfway with her shoulders square and her chin raised.

She stopped ten feet from us and we stopped as well. "Who are you?" she demanded in a clear and superior voice.

"I am Kiyahe and this is Kaya and Neka," Kiyahe introduced us.

"Why are you following us?" she asked, her dark eyes narrowing suspiciously. Her hand twitched and I noticed a pistol in a holster at her side. Kiyahe noticed it as well and his own hand twitched in response.

"We bring a message and a request for your chief. And we deliver it in peace." Kiyahe recited. I had heard him explain our presence three times now and although I was used to the words, my heart gave a start every time, anxious to see people's reactions.

The woman cocked her head to the side while she debated. "Wait here," she said after a few moments, "You move one muscle and your visit will be a short one." She turned her back boldly on us then and walked back to her tribe. The people parted for her and bombarded her with questions. I couldn't see her mouth or hear her voice to know if or what she was telling them.

She returned with two other young men and the chief who wore his headdress. The men also wore sturdy outdoor clothes and had the same looks of guardedness on their faces. I guessed, based on how old they looked and how they shared similar facial features, that the two young men and the woman were siblings and the chief was their father. I also guessed, as the woman was the one doing the talking and standing closest to her father, that she was the oldest and probably the one in line to inherit some type of leadership position someday.

"This is my father, chief of the Navajo, and my brothers. My father has agreed to hear your message and request but asks that you make it short as we have a long way to travel today."

Kiyahe looked to me and I hesitated a moment, waiting for the familiar, subtle howl of the wolf. But the horizon was quiet and after several moments I realized I would not hear my old protector's voice. Perhaps I no longer needed to, now that I was becoming more comfortable and practiced at telling my tale. Before my pausing could become uncomfortable, I stepped forward and launched into my story and the legend.

The woman and her brothers looked to their father after I'd finished, and he looked between each of them and each of us. The silence stretched on as everyone communicated with their eyes until finally the chief spoke. "What do you think, my children?" he asked. Although he asked the question to all his children, his eyes stayed on his daughter and I realized if we were initially rejected I would have to convince her just as much as the chief.

"We don't need their help, we can take care of ourselves," the woman decided. The chief turned to his sons then. The younger looking, scrawny one shrugged nervously, not sure of what answer his father was looking for. The older brother, who looked like a body-building movie star, disagreed with his sister. "I think it's worth considering," he shrugged, the corners of his mouth twitching playfully.

The woman crossed her arms, "We don't know who they are or where they come from, we can't just take their word for it."

"Don't let your pride cloud your eyes, sister," the older brother teased.

"Don't let your hormones cloud yours," she retorted.

My eyes had been following the brother and sister in their conversation, my gaze settling on the bigger brother then, confused by what his sister said. He returned my gaze and boldly winked at me. I tried unsuccessfully to keep from blushing. Kiyahe didn't miss the wink and he stepped closer to me in response. The brother noticed and smiled tauntingly.

"If it would help our case," I said then, eager to bring everyone's attention back to the reason we were there. "I have letters from Chief Cheveyo of the Comanche and Chief Elsu of the Apache. They're proof of where we've been and what alliances we've made."

The chief nodded, "I know Elsu, he is a good friend of mine. I would like to see the letters."

I sighed in relief, glad he wasn't about to base his decision solely on his children's interpretation of us. I gathered that his daughter would have the ultimate say if it came to that, and she didn't seem interested or trusting of us in the slightest.

I pulled the letters out of an inside pocket of my jacket and handed them over. The woman took them from me and handed them to her father. He read them slowly and thoroughly, probably examining them for authenticity. I wondered if he knew what Elsu's handwriting and signature looked like? That was the drawback of using letters to help our case, we couldn't prove we hadn't written them ourselves.

"Ahh, it seems Elsu was not entirely thrilled about pledging his allegiance to you," the chief said.

I nodded, hearing the reluctance in his voice. "Elsu was difficult to convince, I had the support of his people, but I wanted his support as well before continuing on. I won't make a tribe choose between me and their chief. We need to be united. He eventually gave in, but I have to admit he's not our biggest fan."

Although my explanation didn't exactly help my case, it was honest. The chief raised his eyebrows at my explanation and continued to study me with his eyes while his daughter read the letters and then his sons. The daughter pursed her lips as she considered. The brothers merely skimmed the letters, the older one less interested in the papers and more interested in making flirtatious looks at me. I tried to avoid his relentless eye contact, it made me uncomfortable and acutely aware of the quiet tension radiating from Kiyahe. The younger brother was unconcerned with the issue entirely.

"I suppose we will believe you and ally with you as well. At least for now," the chief decided. His daughter wrinkled her nose and nodded, apparently not in agreement with her father but respecting his decision enough not to argue with him. "Now if you'll excuse us, we must get back on the road, and I suggest you not follow us any further," he warned.

"Thank you, sir, and we will not follow you, I promise."

Kiyahe convinced the chief to write a letter of his own testament for us to add to our collection and the chief agreed. It was another short one, stating the basic facts, but the larger our collection of proof, the better. While he wrote the letter, his daughter went back to the tribe to tell them what had happened, her youngest brother following her. The older brother stuck around to continue looking at me in a way that made me blush from embarrassment. While the boy was handsome and strong, he was also immature and almost *too* muscular for my taste.

As soon as we had the letter, we bid the chief goodbye and thanked him for his promise and understanding. As we turned to leave, the older brother quickly and boldly kissed my cheek in parting and Kiyahe pulled me, a little roughly, away as we turned back in the direction of the bus. I stumbled stupidly away with him and the older brother smirked, probably thinking I was stunned at being kissed by such a heart throb. But honestly, I was just shocked that he had had the guts to kiss me and that Kiyahe hadn't thrown a punch at him for doing so.

We made it back to the bus, filled Shilah in on what had happened, and drove off in the western direction. Towards Arizona and the Hopi tribe.

The Hopi were where we expected them to be, on their reservation. They were a small tribe, about the size of ours back at home, and were incredibly welcoming and hospitable. I wondered, after they'd greeted us as if we were old friends, whether the chiefs of larger tribes were more difficult to appeal to because they carried such a large responsibility on their shoulders for so many people.

The Hopi chief was a young man maybe five years older than Kiyahe at the most, and his wife, their shaman, was the most beautiful and kind woman I'd ever met. She was maybe a year older than her husband and seven months pregnant.

"I knew there was a reason for all we'd been through, I just didn't expect that reason to walk up to my front door!" the Hopi chief laughed the first night as we sat by him and his wife around a massive bonfire with the rest of the tribe. His eyes danced in the firelight and his smile was unabashed and youthful. His wife was no less exuberant, and it seemed that their optimism and energy fueled each other and created an aura of happiness that enveloped anyone near them.

The tribe had suffered losses, like all the other tribes we met had, but their chief and shaman had assured them that there was a reason for their suffering and that something good was on the horizon. The chief told us after he'd heard our story that his wife was incredibly intuitive in deciphering the meanings behind her visions and dreams. That she had in fact, predicted our visit more than a week before we'd arrived. They weren't careless in their decision, they did take the time to listen and think about all we told them. But in the end, they accepted our story and promised to ally with us without needing to see any letters or hear how many we had united already.

The first night we sat around the bonfire and, after telling our stories of the disaster and how we'd come to where we were, we listened to dozens of stories from other members of the tribe. Everyone had a story these days and some were more dismal than others, but at the end of each story there was a silence, a moment where we realized we'd made it and that things could only get better from where we were. A moment of gratitude for being spared.

And determination to do something with the life we had left.

We enjoyed our first day and night with the Hopi so much that we promised to spend a little more time with them. The chief promised a big party in our honor for the second night and I was able to convince Kiyahe to let both of the twins accompany us, since we seemed to be very safe with the Hopi tribe. He relented and the four of us returned the next day as the afternoon sun began its decent towards the western horizon.

We wore traditional Native wear the second night, as did the chief, his wife, and a majority of the tribe. At first, I almost didn't recognize the chief and his wife when we arrived at their humble little house; their faces were painted with various patterns in bright blue, white, and yellow. The colors were the colors of the Hopi flag and the symbols were reminiscent of their names and positions within the tribe.

"If you'd like, we could paint your faces too," the chief's wife suggested. I looked to Kiyahe for direction and he shrugged, indifferent to the idea.

"Why not?" I told her. "What better way to fit in, right?"

She laughed and took my hand and led me to their small wooden kitchen table. The paints they had used for their own faces were still sitting out in jars and beginning to dry. She stirred them with a brush while her husband asked Kiyahe and the twins if they wouldn't mind helping him set up tables and chairs. The Hopi chief was not above pitching in and helping out. And, unlike the other chief's we'd met, he had the agility to do so. The boys all looked to me, Kiyahe the only one looking concerned about the idea. I nodded and smiled that he should go. We had nothing to be afraid of here and the thought of having some girl time with no boys around appealed to me.

After the boys had left, the chief's wife asked me to close my eyes as she painted my face in the bright and happy colors of their tribe. The dream I'd had the night before we came to the Hopi was one of my mother putting makeup on my face before my senior prom. It was the only school dance I went to, I was never one for dances as I'd never been asked to go by a boy and I'd never had female friends to encourage me to come with them. My mother had convinced me to go because it was my "last high school dance" and that I would "love it." I had come home before it was half over. The memory of my mother helping me with the makeup was nice and comforting. But of course, like the rest of my dreams, the ending was altered and when I opened my eyes I saw a Native woman, the Hopi shaman, instead of my mother.

We sat in silence at the wobbly wooden table for the first several minutes. The only sounds were of our even breathing, the bustle and voices outside, and the swishing of the wet paint as the chief's wife stirred it and applied it to my face. The paint was warm and slightly sticky. I jerked once or twice, almost falling asleep in the chair.

"So, do you know what you're having?" I asked her, my voice breaking the silence, trying to keep myself awake in the cozy little house.

I could hear the smile in her voice, "A boy," she said with certainty. "I had a dream about him almost two months ago and I know it is a boy." Her confidence in her dreams made me wonder about her other dreams. Especially the one her husband said had predicted my arrival.

"So, you saw me coming over a week ago?" I asked her.

"Yes. I had a dream that a white woman would show up on our door step and ask for our help," she answered softly.

"Did she look like me?"

"Not exactly," the shaman hesitated. "Her face kept changing so I can't remember exactly what she looked like."

"But when I came here you knew it was me. The woman from your dream." I said it as a statement and not a question, but she answered anyway.

"Yes."

"What is it like?" I asked her. "Having visions?"

She sighed and pulled the wet brush away from my face. I opened my eyes to look at her then. She thought it over for a good minute before answering, her eyes not seeing me and her voice far away.

"It's much like having dreams only more…*captivating.* The people and places and events, the *feelings*. At first none of it makes sense. Like a puzzle that's missing pieces. And you *want* it to make sense, you can't explain why, but you just *have* to understand it. You must learn to be patient and to be mindful and perceptive. And when you do, suddenly it all makes sense. It all comes together. Like you've found the missing puzzle pieces on the floor under the table or caught in the corner of the box. Everything comes together, and it makes sense and it's a complete picture."

She paused for a moment. "Does that make any sense?" she laughed.

"It makes perfect sense," I answered, so quietly I almost couldn't hear my own words.

"Why do you ask me about my visions?" she asked then, curiosity and scrutiny visible on her face, even under the paint.

I shrugged, "I don't know, just curiosity I guess. I've never believed in fortune telling or déjà vu or anything so I wonder how it is that you saw me before I saw you."

She pursed her lips, unconvinced. I closed my eyes then and she continued painting my face. The urge to tell her about my strange dreams peaked and I suddenly needed to tell someone. And she seemed like someone I could trust, someone who would understand. I just hoped she wouldn't think I was crazy. Or worse, think me crazy and convince her husband and the tribe not to trust me.

I sighed, "I have…dreams. Strange dreams. I guess that's why I asked." I admitted. I fought the urge to bite my lip and won. She stopped painting and pulled away from me and I worried that I shouldn't've opened my mouth in the first place.

I opened my eyes to her and saw nothing but mild curiosity in her eyes. "And?" she asked. "What are these dreams like?"

I shook my head, trying to put them into words. I was too embarrassed to look at her, so I looked behind her at a clock on the wall as I told her about my dreams before and after I'd found the Potawatomi. The similarities, the differences, everything. The batteries in the clock must have died long ago because the hands didn't move as I spoke, and the glass face was covered in dust.

When I finished she smiled at me and then a tinkling laugh escaped her lips. Her hands, which had been folded gently across her enormously pregnant stomach flew up and clasped in joy. "So interesting! I've never met another shaman before!"

"I'm sorry?" I stammered. The chief's wife smiled from ear to ear, absolutely beaming at me. "No, no, I'm not a shaman. Insane maybe, crazy certainly. But I have no special gift or intuition. I'm just doing what I've been asked to do. It's probably just the stress of it all that's messing with my head," I concluded out loud.

I didn't think it was possible, but the shaman smiled even bigger. "Shaman, medicine woman, call it what you like Kaya. You *are* one! Your dreams, your visions, they're more! So much more! You can't honestly believe that seeing the leaders you've met before you've encountered them is a trick of the mind, can you?! And to see them so clearly, to know what they look like and what their voices sound like, I don't get half the details that you do! It's no wonder you were chosen for this; your gift is very strong indeed. Why I bet..." she babbled on.

"No! Stop! I'm sorry. I shouldn't have told you all this, I should've kept my mouth shut!"

She stopped talking and her smile shrank but didn't entirely disappear off her face. "I'm sorry," she apologized. "It's just so exciting for me to meet..." she started again, but I gave her a warning look and she stopped. She took a breath and tried to be serious, although the smile only seemed to grow on her beautiful face. "I know this seems shocking and maybe a little scary for you but it's not, it's an amazing blessing, I promise you."

"I'm not a shaman," I told her sternly. "The tribe I've joined already has a shaman anyways." I didn't tell her that Kiyahe's mother, Nakoma, was losing her connection to the spirit world or the ancestors or wherever it was that her visions came from. I realized that it would only encourage the idea that this Hopi shaman was already convinced was true.

"It sounds unconventional, yes," she agreed. "But so much that we didn't expect to occur has already happened. You can't deny that the Great Spirit has given you much more than you bargained for already," she pointed out. I had nothing to say to that and she returned to painting my face, letting me absorb the possibility.

"I'll consider the idea, but will you promise me one thing?" I asked her. I couldn't look into her eyes to communicate my sincerity or evaluate hers because she was painting my eyelids at that moment.

"Yes?" she asked.

"Can we keep this to ourselves for now? My tribe's shaman is Kiyahe's mother and I don't want to freak him out with the idea of all this."

She painted silently for a few seconds, considering.

"Kiyahe is the son of your tribe's chief and shaman?" she asked.

"Yes."

More silence.

"I promise not to say anything while you are all here."

When she pulled away I looked at her and thought she looked sincere.

But later that night I realized the conviction in her words.

She had promised not to say anything while we were visiting, but that didn't mean she wouldn't say anything to her husband or the tribe *after* we left.

And worse.

She'd gathered that Kiyahe's lineage would make him the next chief of our tribe. And if she believed I had visions…

Ahh hell.

We do not walk alone. Great Being walks beside us. Know this and be grateful.

–Polingaysi Qoyawayma, Hopi.

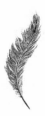

Chapter Six

I tried to bury the idea in my head that I might be a shaman. And at first, it worked.

The Hopi chief's wife didn't say anything more to me about it that night and the party was especially distracting and invigorating. Between the music, dancing, conversation, and laughter, there was more than enough to entertain my mind.

But when we got back to the bus, exhausted from the enjoyable night with the Hopi, everyone went straight to bed, and I was left alone with my thoughts. I considered and reconsidered the meaning and purpose behind my dreams until at some point I was completely enveloped in one.

In the dream I was back in Atlantis, my hometown, walking down the street in the dark on Halloween. I had gotten off work late at Julio's Supermarket and I had had to walk home in the cold because my car was in the local mechanic's shop with engine problems. My parents had debated whether to go to the costume party at my dad's boss's house and I had convinced them that I would be fine to walk home alone. I was seventeen, after all, and I knew the town like the back of my hand.

Despite the hour and the absence of moonlight, I could see fairly well with the dim street lights, the distant porch lights that had been left on for trick-or-treaters, and the soft glow from carved pumpkins. I was not afraid, just cold and in a hurry to get home.

If the dream had stayed true to the memory, I would have made it home just fine. I would have come in the house, turned off the porch light, closed the curtains, locked the doors, taken a warm shower, and gone to bed.

But the dream became more than a memory and this one had the most terrifying ending I had experienced yet.

I was walking down the street again, alone in the cold darkness. And as I walked the small but comforting lights from the street corners and houses dimmed. I walked faster in response, beginning to feel the first inkling of fear. As the lights diminished into blackness, I began to run, adrenaline and panic coursing through me. When I was completely surrounded by pitch black darkness, I stopped running. Listening for cars or people or anything to give me a sense of direction.

But all was silent.

I whirled around in one spot, unable to see, unable to hear. But I could feel. I could feel the cold air, I could feel the hair on my arms standing on end. And something else…. a presence. I stood still focusing on the one sensation I had left. Someone or something was with me in the dark.

There were hands then, from a person. Large strong hands, probably a man's hands, I had to guess. Who's they were, I did not know, and the uncertainty made me freeze as the hands touched me. They started caressing me, brushing my face, my arms, and I began to squirm away from them because I didn't know who it was that was touching me. And then they became rough; groping, scratching, pulling. I slapped at the hands and tried to run but I couldn't find my feet. I tried to scream but I couldn't find my voice. That was when the hands, or the person behind the hands, became angry.

The hands started slapping and punching me, each blow taking me off guard because I couldn't see where it was coming from or guess where it would hit me. The hands pulled my hair, slapped my face, punched my torso, scratched my skin. And then they were around my throat, constricting, suffocating. I fought and beat against them, but they were too strong. I couldn't tell if I was blacking out because everything was black already. I let myself go limp then, not in defeat but in manipulation. I wanted the hands to think I was dead and let go of me.

And then I heard a deafening blast and lurched up in bed.

۾

It was still dark but there was just enough pallid moonlight filtering through the blinds that I could make out my bedroom in the bus. I gasped and clutched my throat; the ghost of the hands was still there. The only sounds in the room were my frantic breathing and ringing ears. I listened for another blast but heard nothing. Eventually my pulse returned to normal and the ringing in my ears stopped. I could hear Kiyahe snoring softly beyond the door to the bunkroom. Surely the blast must have been in my dream or he would've woken up. I laid down in bed again and waited for dawn, this dream was the scariest one yet. A nightmare more than a dream. I thought about what the Hopi shaman had said about my dreams being visions

I couldn't help but briefly compare him to Kiyahe. They looked equally strong, in fact I really couldn't say who would win in a fight if they ever got into a physical one. And they were equally good looking, too. But they were good looking in different ways. Kiyahe was handsome and dignified where this man was sexy and seductive. And their eyes, their eyes were the biggest difference between them. Kiyahe's were a brilliant, captivating blue that made me feel safe and cared for where this man's were a deep obsidian that made me feel entranced and impish.

I didn't realize until Kiyahe introduced us that I had moved so that I was partially hidden behind Kiyahe's right side. The man didn't look at Neka or I and I was glad for that because something about him intimidated me. The man introduced himself as Kalona and demanded to know our intentions immediately. He did not shout or threaten, but his tone was brisk and his sentences were curt. Kiyahe told him no more than the general purpose behind our visit and Kalona revealed no more than what he was specifically asked. We came to a standoff, he and his friends watching us and us watching them. I wanted to speak up, but I was afraid to draw Kalona's attention to me. Would he become angry at being addressed by a white woman outsider? Or would he notice my weak-kneed interest in him and use it to his advantage?

When it was clear we weren't leaving, he jerked his chin at us and turned to take us to their chief. We followed; Kiyahe in the lead, me following, and Neka taking up the rear. Kalona's friends followed closely behind us.

The Miwok people did not treat us any differently than the other tribes had. Even so, I felt more on edge. My increased discomfort and anxiety stemmed from the nightmare I'd had before we'd arrived and the hostility that Kalona and his friends exuded. I fervently hoped that Kalona wasn't the chief's son, I did not want to have to convince him of our goal. I worried that if he so much as made eye contact with me when it was my turn to speak that I would run away or melt into a puddle on the ground.

The chief lived in a squalid little house at the top of a dune at the northernmost edge of the reservation. Kalona and his friends led us inside, having already informed the chief of our arrival beforehand. The chief was an elderly man who was very ill. He sat in a worn leather chair that was in scarcely better shape than he was. His head and hands shook slightly as he sat there, and Kalona occasionally helped him sit up straighter in his chair as he was too weak to keep himself upright. His hair was almost completely translucent, the strands countable, and his eyes were milky and sunken in his head. The liveliest thing about him was his cough which racked his whole body and was so violent at times that I was afraid a lung would end up in his lap. He had to take several moments after each fit to regain his raspy breath. I couldn't help but pity him, this man didn't have much time left.

Kiyahe requested that their shaman be present, but Kalona spoke for the chief and informed us that the chief's wife had died long ago and that they had been without a shaman ever since.

"And what is your purpose here?" Kiyahe asked Kalona.

Kalona's eyes narrowed but he answered calmly and confidently. "I am the next in line to become chief."

"I see," Kiyahe said casually. "So, you are the chief's son?"

"No," Kalona answered, albeit with a touch of bitterness. "The chief and his wife never had any children. I was chosen." The words sounded as if Kalona was proud of it too. As if being chosen was an even greater honor than being born for the job.

Kiyahe turned to me then and motioned that I should speak. I had been dreading the idea but now I had no choice. I glanced at Kalona and his friends and felt my knees shake under their glares. I locked my knees and focused on the chief instead, who was much less intimidating. I thought I heard the faint howl of a wolf before I started.

When I finished there was absolute silence.

Then Kalona started shouting.

"YOU'RE LYING, YOU ALL ARE! JUST WHO DO YOU THINK YOU ARE THAT YOU CAN COME HERE AND DEMAND THIS OF US?! GET OUT, NOW!"

Kalona's deafening voice filled the room and even though we were less than ten feet apart, he closed the distance between he and I in less than three strides. Kiyahe intercepted him before he could get in front of my face and the two stood toe-to-toe in front of me. Kalona kept shouting and Kiyahe struggled to keep his calm as he tried to talk him down. Kalona's friends moved to flank him and Neka stepped forward as well. I gently but quickly grabbed Kiyahe's right hand, which was clenched into a fist and shaking, with both of my hands. The chief tried to demand silence, but his faint voice was drowned out by all the talking and shouting.

"STOP!" I shouted at Kalona. He and everyone else was silenced by my outburst. His fury was turned on me and I had to look at everyone but him to escape the heat of his gaze. "I think the chief wants to say something and we're being disrespectful."

Everyone took a step back then and looked to the chief. He smiled in thanks to me and spoke in between coughs then. "A good chief considers all sides before he makes such a decision. I would like to see the letters you've mentioned, and I would like to consult with Kalona before making a decision. But first I must pray and rest. Please come back tonight as our honored guests, I promise an answer for you soon. Kalona my boy, take me to bed."

I was grateful for the chief's consideration but more so for his need for Kalona's help to get out of the chair and to his bedroom. It kept Kalona's hands and attention busy as we left. His friends, however, followed us all the way back to the edge of the reservation. They knew what general direction we had left in and I didn't have to ask Kiyahe twice to move the bus to a different spot.

When we had wondered if the Apache were a threat, Kiyahe had suggested it might not be safe to go back to them. We had argued over it then and Kiyahe had admitted he cared for me, enough to throw away our progress to keep me safe. That argument had ended in my favor, we went back to the Apache and gained them as another ally.

We argued that same argument again over the Miwok and, once again, I won. We would go back to them that night even though it was a risk to my safety and even though Kiyahe didn't like it.

The walk back to the Miwok reservation was longer because we'd moved the bus an extra mile south and a half mile east. We still came in at the same spot we had before though, so that no one would know we'd moved our camp. As we'd expected, Kalona's friends were waiting at the edge of the reservation for us. Once again, they demanded we give up our weapons, once again Kiyahe refused, and once again they ran to get Kalona before letting us through.

Kalona seemed to have calmed down during the few hours that we were gone, and I was glad for that. It would be hard enough looking at him or talking to him without a fiery rage directed at me. He greeted us with a serene face and smooth voice that melted like chocolate. I allowed a small smile in my greeting, hoping he could be encouraged to change his mind about us. Kiyahe, of course, wasn't nearly as cordial. He stayed within centimeters of me and never took his hardened blue eyes off Kalona's liquid black ones. His hand lingered on his grandfather's pistol, which was now in a visible holster at his side. I'd noticed him make the change at the bus, before we'd come back to the reservation. The look in his eyes had dissuaded me from even attempting to argue about where he kept his pistol.

The rest of the Miwok, with the encouragement of their chief, greeted us and treated us with respect and hospitality. Some of the more extroverted ones approached us, welcomed us, and introduced us. The chief mustered as much enthusiasm and energy as he could and maneuvered about with the assistance of a cane, smiling and talking with everyone. He greeted Kiyahe and Neka with surprisingly strong handshakes and a warm embrace for me. My fear of how the Miwok would perceive us began to wane and I let myself relax just a little around the tribe.

The feast in the Miwok meeting lodge was grand and fulfilling. It gave me the strength I needed to repeat my story and the legend to the people. I kept most of my eye contact on the people, who's expressions could only be described as considering. Like their chief, they would chew the idea over and take their time in deciding what to make of it. I chanced a glance at the chief and Kalona who sat at the head table with us. The chief was listening politely, still considering. Kalona's expression was blank and unreadable.

The chief announced to us and the tribe that he would like more time to pray to the Great Spirit and convene with the future chief about whether to promise allegiance with us or not. He explained that without a shaman to help interpret what the will of the Great Spirit would be in the matter, he would like to meditate and pray for guidance.

"I will also be more confident in my decision after I've read what the other chiefs have to say about Kaya in their letters and after Kalona and I are on the same page."

I had nothing to hide or worry about with the letters, I had read them myself almost half a dozen times each and although some were more enthusiastic about being allies than others, all had come to the same conclusion thus far. But I worried about Kalona and the chief being on the same page. If them being on the same page didn't earn us another alliance, I didn't know what we would do.

The chief disbanded the meeting then but encouraged the tribe to stay and get to know Kiyahe, Neka, and I at the fire pit. The massive brick-laid fire pit was below the dunes, down on the beach, several hundred yards behind the lodge building. As twenty or so people cleaned up the lodge where we'd eaten, well over a hundred people headed to the fire pit on the beach, the boys and I included. A dozen men and boys gathered driftwood on the beach and piled it high in the massive pit. When they set it aflame, it glowed in various shades of blue and green from the sea salt. It grew dark very quickly then and the towering glow of the fire illuminated a large circumference around it, including all the people. Everything outside the ring of that glow was hidden in dark shadows.

I socialized with people of all ages for well over an hour before Kalona approached me. Kiyahe and Neka, who had given me some space while I talked with others, moved to my sides immediately and watched Kalona with distrusting eyes. Kalona held his hands out in surrender and it reminded me of the times when Kiyahe had made the same gesture when we'd entered other reservations. Something about it was different though, with Kiyahe it was purely in defense. With Kalona and his sly smile, it was almost taunting. An invitation. A dare.

"I would just like to apologize to Kaya," Kalona purred. His voice made me shiver it was so beautiful, just like the rest of him. He held out his hand for me to shake and before I could accept or reject it, Kiyahe stepped in between us, his body blocking my view of Kalona.

I peered around Kiyahe's shoulder, worried that his reaction would set Kalona off again, but instead Kalona smiled, exposing his pearly white teeth. Although he was facing away from the fire, his eyes danced with light. "How can I make amends if your protector won't let me?" The silky, slightly teasing words were directed at me, but Kalona did not take his eyes off Kiyahe when he spoke.

"You don't need to touch her for her to hear you. Say what you need to say and be done with it," Kiyahe growled.

I put a hand on his arm to calm him, but he kept glaring at Kalona who appeared calm and comfortable. I gently grabbed Kiyahe's chin and tugged until he tore his eyes away from Kalona to look at me. "A handshake isn't going to hurt me, and you'll be right here with me," I said calmly.

"I don't trust him," he whispered fiercely, low enough that Kalona couldn't hear him. "And I don't want him touching you."

I ignored the second comment, it was filled with jealousy and I wasn't sure at that moment how to address it. I responded to the first instead, "You never trust anybody, how are we going get others to trust us if we can't do the same for them? We have to give him a chance to change his mind, his opinion is important to the chief's decision."

He opened his mouth to disagree, then closed it, then opened it again, trying to think of a response against what I had said. I added to my resolve before he could argue further. "And not only is his opinion important now but it will be vital in the future when he's chief. Which could be very soon." I didn't have to point out the Miwok chief's delicate health, Kiyahe would have to be blind not to see it and know what it meant for us.

His shoulders slumped in acquiescence and he turned to face Kalona, who's smile was full of charm.

Kiyahe nodded his allowance with a stern face and stood ever so slightly to the side, the length of his arm touching mine from shoulder to wrist. I tried to ignore the heat and electricity of his touch and focus on the future chief. Kalona couldn't have heard what we said but his eyes looked either pleased or amused at our obvious quarrel. I hoped he was just being ornery and not overly observant of the tension between my protector and I. We seriously needed to get a grip on our bickering.

Kalona apologized profusely to me, explaining that he was under a lot of pressure and stress in being chosen as the next chief. The current chief, whom he thought of as a father, was very old and in poor health and it hurt Kalona to see him so fragile. And in such perilous times, with the fate of their tribe unknown, the stress of everything had gotten to Kalona and he had unfairly dumped his emotions on me. I believed him sincere, especially as he continued on worrying about his predecessor who he said had practically raised him.

The autumn air began to reach me even through my jacket and after a few shivers, he invited me to sit next to him by the fire so that I would be warmer. He was respectful, not daring to touch me and not taunting or teasing Kiyahe who followed me as if we were handcuffed. He and the boys sat cross-legged in the sand on either side of me and I tucked my legs up under me as I was wearing a buckskin dress. Kalona told me his life story by the fire, about his alcoholic father who left when he was eight and his drug-addicted mother who died of an overdose when he was twelve. The chief and his wife had taken him in when his mother died and then the chief's wife had died of ovarian cancer just two years later. He and the chief had become inseparable after that. I couldn't relate to having such a tumultuous childhood, but my heart still gave out to him for what he had been through. I put a hand on his arm in comfort, his godly handsomeness forgotten in the human honesty of his past. Kiyahe sucked in a breath and I quickly pulled away. I let my hair fall in my face while my blush cooled, I was a sucker for people with sob stories and my instant reaction when I heard them was to comfort and try to make everything better. Kalona smiled sheepishly in thanks for my effort and in silent apology for upsetting my protector. He continued telling me about his teen years and how much hell he'd given the chief during them.

"I realized after I blew up on you at the house that I haven't been controlling my emotions as well as I'd thought. I've really just been bottling them up and I'm sorry for unleashing them on you."

I accepted his apology for the dozenth time and suffocated my desire to reach for him again. The man I had met this afternoon and the man who was sitting next to me now seemed like completely different people. I liked this version of Kalona, the humble, honest version.

We talked about trivial things then, the topics much lighter, and before long I found myself laughing and smiling. For a moment I felt guilty for spending so much time talking to Kalona instead of everyone else but then I remembered that he was practically a chief and that it was important to have his support. Plus, I was genuinely enjoying myself and I thought I deserved just a taste of that.

We talked into the night, oblivious to the dwindling numbers around us. When Kiyahe finally interrupted to suggest that we call it a night, I realized how very tired I was. The four of us stood and as I told Kalona goodnight, he suddenly reached for my hand and kissed it. I stared at him, dumbstruck, as he turned to leave.

He didn't make it five steps before Kiyahe grabbed him roughly by the shoulder and tried to whip him back around. Kalona really only turned halfway around, he was strong and quite possibly ready for Kiyahe to make such a move.

"How dare you touch her!" Kiyahe shouted.

Neka jumped in between them, his left hand on Kiyahe's chest, pushing him back, his right hand ready to shove against Kalona if necessary. But Kalona didn't move, he just glared angrily at Kiyahe in warning, keeping his temper in check. Kiyahe clenched his fists and I lurched forward, grabbing his biceps with my hands and tugging back. His fists unclenched at my touch, but he didn't move back. His eyes blazed in fury.

"Kiyahe stop it, it's fine. Stop it!" I shouted at him in fear and anger.

The few Miwok men and women who had lingered that late were staring openmouthed at the four of us. The men looked ready to jump in, hopefully to stop a fight and not to join it. A blush of embarrassment and anger blazed up my neck and across my face. We looked like children in a squabble, not mature adult leaders. Talk of the incident would spread like wildfire by tomorrow morning.

"We need to leave, and you need to cool off," I said sternly. Kiyahe pulled his arms out of my grasp then and stalked off, back up the beach towards the lodge. I apologized to Kalona first, who dismissed the reaction as nothing and then I apologized to the bystanders before turning to follow Kiyahe. Neka followed me back up the beach, up the dune, and out of the reservation back towards the bus. He didn't say anything as we powerwalked to catch up with Kiyahe. Or if he did, I didn't hear him through the roaring argument playing out in my head that I knew I was about to get into with Kiyahe.

Be tolerant of those who are lost on their path. Ignorance, conceit, anger, jealousy, and greed stem from a lost soul. Pray that they will find guidance.

—Native American quote.

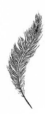

Chapter Seven

I didn't sleep well that night. Partly because of my recurring nightmare and partly because Kiyahe and I had gotten into a two-hour shouting match before bed. The twins had escaped to the bunk room to give us our privacy and dodge the verbal bullets Kiyahe and I were firing at each other in the main compartment of the bus. In summary: Kiyahe accused me of being careless and too trusting and I accused him of being jealous and hot-headed.

To make matters worse, the chief fell ill the next day with pneumonia and his healer refused to let us see or speak to him until she was sure he wasn't contagious. Kalona picked up the roll of 'temporary chief' with ease and was our constant escort as we spent time with the Miwok.

We helped them rebuild, repair, and renew their reservation as well as hunt and fish for food to keep everyone fed. As the days went by, being with the Miwok people became more enjoyable. Kalona's initial outburst was all but forgotten and he and I reached the point where we were shamelessly friendly with each other. And I enjoyed his company and friendship. As much as I wanted to keep moving, I was genuinely enjoying myself with the Miwok and their young chief-to-be. After a few days, Neka allowed himself to enjoy our time with them too. Kiyahe never did reach the point of enjoyment but he did gradually become less possessive and more accepting.

Two weeks later, the chief had recovered enough for us to see him and he told us that he had decided to ally his tribe with ours and all the others we had allied with. It was a relief to everyone and, of course, we had a banquet and party to celebrate. The celebration took place on Halloween night, making the occasion even more festive.

Drinks flowed freely as Kalona and his friends ran the music, using car batteries to power speakers and stereo systems. Before long, the beach area around the roaring fire pit was crowded, everyone swaying and laughing as they danced to the upbeat tempo of the music. Shadows flitted across the walls of the dunes as people danced all around. Neka and I gave ourselves to the thrill of the party and when it appeared that Kalona would be kept occupied as the DJ of the night, Kiyahe gave in to the party as well.

The older men and women and the young children were the first to leave but a good one hundred people or so remained on the beach with us after nearly two hours. The night was unseasonably warm on the coast and with all the dancing and mingling that I was doing, I drank as often as I became thirsty. After a couple hours, several of the partiers were visibly drunk and Kiyahe, Neka, and I were quite buzzed from the quenching alcohol. At the end of the song, "Roll Up" by Fitz & The Tantrums, I excused myself to go refill my plastic cup and to cool down.

I had almost entirely forgotten about Kalona when he met me at the tables where pre-mixed drinks sat on top and coolers with bottles and cans sat underneath. I sheepishly looked at his face instead of his torso, which was once again shirtless.

"Can I get you a refill?" he asked with a crooked smile that set my already pounding heart into overdrive. I nodded impishly and let my hair fall partially over my features to hide the blush that was warming my already flushed face. I had thought that being around him so much in the last two weeks would make me immune to his looks and charm, but it hadn't. In fact, getting to know him as I had was making it harder to be around someone so amazing when I felt so plain myself. He mixed Sangria and fruit punch in my cup, making it a little stronger than I wanted, and handed it to me. I sipped slowly from it, trying to slake my thirst without worsening my intoxication. We stood together at the table watching the partiers in silence. Neka was putting the charm on a girl who clearly wasn't going to give him the time of day and I shook my head and smiled.

When I caught sight of Kiyahe, I noticed that a young woman had approached and started a conversation with him in my absence. She appeared to be a year or two older than Kiyahe and was heart wrenchingly beautiful. Her long, glossy black hair hung down to the small of her back and her red cotton dress hugged her every curve. The firelight illuminated her flawless bronze skin and glinted off her perfect white teeth as she smiled and laughed. She was older, more voluptuous, and far more confident than I would ever be. I felt like a gangly fifteen-year-old just looking at her. I watched them carefully as they talked and felt a twinge of pride that Kiyahe did not appear especially interested in her. Just as I was taking a sip of my drink and working up the courage to approach them, she took Kiyahe's hand and pulled him into the crowd as a slow song started.

I inhaled my drink in surprise and choked and sputtered embarrassingly. Kalona took the cup from me before I could spill it, setting it on the table with one hand and thumping my back with the other hand.

"Whoa there, you alright?" he chuckled.

"Sorry, yeah I'm fine," I rasped between coughs. My eyes darted across the dancers until I found Kiyahe and the girl dancing in the crowd. My satisfaction of Kiyahe's indifference instantly disappeared. The woman was still laughing and smiling and now Kiyahe was too. A new flush spread across my face, neck, and collarbone and the flicker of jealousy fueled its warmth. Part of me wanted to march over to them and separate them with my own two hands while the other part of me wanted to close my eyes and pretend nothing was happening.

"… we don't have to if you don't want to. I just thought it's so nice out and that maybe you could use a break from the party," Kalona was saying. I turned around stupidly.

"I'm sorry, what? I wasn't paying attention." I fought the urge to look back at Kiyahe and the girl. Suddenly the gorgeous guy in front of me mattered little compared to my soul-bound, life-long protector who was completely oblivious to my absence.

I forced my eyes and ears to focus on Kalona as he repeated his request to go on a walk with me. I hesitated for a second, part of me was afraid to leave Kiyahe alone with his dance partner and the other part of me wanted to get as far away from them as possible. Cowardly, I chose the latter and let Kalona escort me away from the party.

He held out his arm for me like a gentleman and I took it more for necessity than flattery. The alcohol was still running through me and the rocky beach was not exactly easy to maneuver through. We walked the length of two football fields away from the glow of the party and through the shadows to a small grove of palm trees, bent towards the water from years of standing against the wind. I inhaled the cool, salty air and leaned against the trunk of one of the trees, enjoying the undiluted sound of the waves as they gently caressed the shore with each surge. Kalona kept me actively engaged in conversation and I was able to forget about Kiyahe and the girl for just a little while.

"So where do you go after this?" Kalona asked quietly, kicking at the dirt with his shoe. I cocked my head to the side, surprised at the question. No one had asked where we were going yet, only where we had been. "Uhm…Washington I think. To the Spokane tribe."

Kalona stopped kicking the dirt and looked up at me then, pain twisting his beautiful features. I pushed off the tree and stepped towards him without thinking, putting my hand on his arm. "What's wrong?" I whispered.

He hesitated before confessing. "I don't want you to leave. Not yet anyway."

Without thinking I removed my hand from his arm and took a step back, not sure what to say to that. For a second, I worried that my reaction would upset Kalona, but then he took a step towards me, closing the small distance I had just created. He took both of my hands in his and I stared at him stupidly with my mouth hanging open.

"I really like you Kaya," he said softly, his voice like smooth honey, the warmth of it caressing my face. And before I could begin to form a coherent thought, he put his mouth to mine and kissed me.

It was my first kiss and the reality of it shocked me like a taser. For several seconds all I could do was stand there and let his mouth move against mine. But as soon as the rusty gears in my head were able to turn again, I pulled away. I did not want this. This was wrong.

In another life I would have swooned and melted in the arms of someone like Kalona. But then and there I could not deny that this was not what I wanted. That *he* was not what I wanted. My thoughts flew the couple hundred yards back down the beach to the one I really wanted and couldn't have. To my protector.

"Uhm…We should go…I shouldn't be here…" the half intelligible responses stumbled out of my mouth as I turned to leave.

And then a rough, hot hand grabbed my shoulder and whipped me back around.

My stomach dropped and my heart stopped beating.

Kalona's large, calloused hands gripped my arms just above my elbows so hard that it hurt.

"Let me go!" I warned him, trying to sound commanding instead of pleading. I tried to squirm out of his grasp, but he only gripped me tighter and shook me, rattling my brain.

"What's the matter Kaya? Need to ask for your protector's permission first?" Kalona taunted, his black eyes glinting in the moonlight, a smug smile on his lips.

His words and the arrogant look on his face lit me with anger and I glared at him, this was not the Kalona I had come to know. This was the Kalona who had exploded in anger the first day we met. But my glare didn't deter him, it only egged him on. He yanked me to him and kissed me again.

I turned my face away from his kiss and started to thrash in his iron-like grip, managing to break my right arm free, although I nearly ripped it from my socket in the process. His smile disappeared just before my fist connected with his jaw.

I didn't regret the punch.

Until he came after me.

He snatched my arm back with long fingers before I could throw another punch and he twisted it, pinning my arm like a chicken wing behind my back. He shoved me into the palm tree I had been leaning on earlier and the bark smashed into my chest. The impact knocked the wind out of me.

Darkness toyed with my vision at the edge of my peripherals. A flicker of my nightmare ran through my head.

As I gasped for air, Kalona pulled me down to the sand with him and rolled me over so that he was on top of me. His weight pinned me solidly to the beach and he pinned my wrists above my head. I started to scream for help, for Kiyahe, when the sudden sting of a slap took the words right out of my mouth.

"Shut up or I'll kill you!" Kalona growled in my ear. My head screamed in astonishment and fear, 'My nightmare! Kiyahe isn't here! I'm all alone!' That's when I felt cold metal press up against my jugular. I couldn't look down to see it, but I knew he had pulled a knife on me then. One of his hands held my wrists above my head while the other held the knife against my throat. He dragged the blade from the base of my throat to the collar of my dress, a deep cut oozing blood as he went. I screamed from the pain, unable to stop myself. Then he started to cut at my clothes, cutting into my arms, legs, and torso in the process.

"You think you can come here and take whatever you want?! That everyone will bow down to you like some kind of queen?! This is *my* tribe and you will *not* take it from me! I will not bow down to *anyone*. *Especially* not you!" Kalona hissed in my ear.

He kept on spewing threats and insults and in his spiel, he brought his head down by my ear so I could hear every word clearly. That's when I made my move, turning my head and latching onto his ear with my teeth. I bit down as hard as I could, tasting the metallic tang of blood, and I threw my knee into his back. He howled as he rolled off of me and as soon as his weight left me, I rolled sideways away from him and scrambled up to run.

I screamed with everything in me as I ran towards the glow of the fire and the shadows of the partiers as they mingled around it. No one turned to see me running towards them, the music was too loud, and it drowned out my screams. I was almost forty yards from the ring of light when a weight crashed into me and arms locked around my middle as I was tackled like a football player.

Kalona pinned me under him again but this time both of his hands were wrapped around my neck, cutting off my air and screams. He'd given up on raping me. Now he simply meant to kill me. I feebly tried to pull his hands off my throat and noticed that the knife was not in them. I sprawled my arms and legs around in the sand, feeling for the knife. Just before the blackness claimed the last spots in my vision, my right hand bumped the cold metal in the sand. I grasped it and fell limp, letting Kalona think he'd killed me. As soon as his hands left my throat, I lurched up and plunged the knife into his left side, driving it in as far as it would go.

Everything slowed, both of our faces were plastered in shock, both of us panting heavily. Kalona looked at the knife sticking out of his side. I watched in horror as he grabbed it and pulled it out. It dripped with his blood and scarlet stained his bronze skin where the wound was. He turned his eyes to me then and they were no longer shocked but blazing with fury. He was still positioned on top of me, with the knife in hand again.

Time resumed with furious speed then. Kalona raised his right hand with the knife to stab me.

A deafening blast, so loud that my ears screamed in protest.

Warm droplets spattered my face.

And Kalona fell off of me, a second wound, a bullet wound, in the bicep of the arm with the knife.

I floundered backwards, away from him. I whipped my head around to see Kiyahe aiming a familiar pistol at my attacker, a faint wisp of smoke whirling away from the barrel. He, and Neka behind him, were staring at my attacker laying in the sand. Kalona wasn't dead though, not yet. We could all hear his loud gasping from where he laid. I'd never seen Kiyahe's face so enraged and twisted with pain before. His right hand, holding the pistol, shook slightly in fury. As if he'd like to shoot Kalona a few more times. Neka just stared at Kalona in shock.

"Kiyahe," I whimpered, the fear of what had just happened and the pain of my wounds taking my last bit of strength. Both boys turned to look at me then. I quickly and clumsily tried to stand and run to Kiyahe, wanting nothing more than to have him hold me, but he made it to me before I could get my feet underneath me. He dropped to the sand beside me, leaving his grandfather's pistol in the sand beside him and pulled me into his arms. He commanded Neka to go tell the chief what had happened and as Neka turned to leave, I broke down in tears and let Kiyahe rock me like a child.

As we waited for the chief and Neka to return, Kiyahe and I apologized over a dozen times to each other.

"I'm so sorry Marie. I thought you were safe with Neka and then that girl told me she was Kalona's cousin and as soon as she said his name, I started looking everywhere for you. I will never let you out of my sight again, Marie, I swear it. I am so, so sorry."

"No, I'm sorry, Kiyahe. I'm such an idiot for letting him draw me away like that and I'll never go off without you again."

My attacker moaned in the sand then, pools of blood soaking into the beach by his left side and right arm. Kiyahe glared at him as if he'd like to finish him off but I turned his face to me instead and continued blubbering my apologies to him.

The chief and Neka came back with two men, two women, and a stretcher. The men were not Kalona's friends and I was grateful for that, I didn't want to risk any more fights that night. As the men loaded Kalona onto the stretcher and one of the women tended to him, the other woman tended to me and the chief apologized profusely to me on behalf of his almost-son.

"He is troubled, that I have always known. But it is no excuse. I just hoped that with my love and teaching, he could rise above his past, but now I see that I was wrong. I am so terribly sorry for what has happened here, and I pray that his actions have not tainted your view of our people. I sincerely wish to be allied with you and the other tribes."

We took a roundabout route to the edge of the reservation, avoiding the partygoers. And the chief walked with us, apologizing the whole way. I worried about what this new stress would do to his health and I continued telling him that as long as Kalona was not made chief of their tribe, our friendship was still intact. It was an easy agreement for him to make. We left on as good a note as possible, considering the circumstances.

Back at the bus, Neka and Shilah gave us our privacy by going outside to pack up our camp. I knew Neka would tell Shilah about the attack, and I couldn't be upset about that. Even if I wanted to pretend it had never happened, I couldn't because I had walked into the bus covered in sand, blood, wounds, and the remaining tatters of my dress. The nice thing about the twins, though, is that I knew they wouldn't bring it up in front of me.

Kiyahe gently guided me with his hand on the small of my back to my bedroom. I convinced him I was ok to dress myself and he waited patiently outside the bedroom door until I was ready.

Kalona didn't manage to take from me what he wanted but he certainly left his marks. My arms, legs, and torso were covered in gashes from the knife and bluish black bruises from his fist. My chest, the space between my breasts, was purple from colliding with the tree and I could still taste his bitter blood in my mouth. The feeling of his hands around my throat was still there. Everything felt battered, but it was nothing compared to the ache in my heart.

As amazing as he made himself out to be, I wasn't in love with Kalona. Not even close. But to know that I had trusted him as a friend and future ally, that's what smarted. There were warning signs right from the beginning that he was dangerous, my nightmares being one of them, but like Kiyahe had said, I was too trusting. Too willing to see a change of heart that wasn't there. I mentally slapped myself for being so stupid and careless. God knew I would be far more careful from then on.

And what hurt even more than what Kalona had done to me or what I had gotten myself into, was that it had hurt Kiyahe as well. He'd warned me, and I didn't listen to him. He'd cared for me and I threw that care to the side. I swore to myself (again) that I wouldn't make his job any harder for him than it already was. I had learned my lesson. And I hoped he wouldn't beat himself up too hard in learning his.

Kiyahe sat on the bed with me while we talked about what had happened. At first, I didn't want to think about it, didn't even want to acknowledge what had transpired. But Kiyahe told me that talking it out would help me feel better. And in an emotional sense, it did.

Kiyahe covered me in bandages to keep my cuts from re-opening and I took aspirin before crawling under the covers. I didn't have to ask Kiyahe to stay with me that night, or any other night after that. He slept alongside me from then on. We still hadn't figured out our relationship, what we could be or what we were to each other. Right then and there though, we were cemented together as protector and leader. That bond was allowed and was now stronger than it had ever been before.

Our first teacher is our own heart.

—Cheyenne.

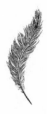

Chapter Eight

We left the Miwok area first thing in the morning, but we didn't rush to Washington in one day. We stopped in Oregon, the boys allowing me some time to heal physically and emotionally before we met the Spokane tribe. Unfortunately, I couldn't take more than a few days to do so. We were behind schedule and we had to keep moving.

I not only learned to trust in Kiyahe more, but also to trust in my dreams. I had another confusing, but good dream the night before we met the Spokane tribe and sure enough, they were friendly and welcoming to us when we arrived. We helped their tribe during the time their leaders and elders took to deliberate our proposal. There wasn't much to repair as far as the reservation went, they were well protected from the meteor shower as their reservation was nestled in the middle of one of the massive forests of the Olympic area. We soon learned that more of their people had survived than any other tribe besides our own. Our safety was in the legend, theirs in their forests. I was reminded again of how the damage of the disaster had been more concentrated on civilization and that most of nature had survived and flourished afterwards. Those people, living so close to nature, were mostly spared.

But even so, their tribe population was, and had been, only around 200 people, one of the smallest we'd encountered. With minimal damage to their reservation, we helped them hunt and fish instead, trying to keep those 200 well fed and to stock up for the winter. The rain, combined with the chill of autumn, reminded me that the cold season was not far off. I prayed that God or the Great Spirit or

A few days after we arrived on their reservation, the Spokane people came to the same conclusion as the other tribes and joined our alliance. There was another party, but this time Kiyahe stayed close to me and I to him.

We drove out of Washington, across Idaho, and into the rugged, rocky state of Montana to the Crow tribe. They were one of the larger tribes we'd met and, unlike the Spokane, their reservation sat out in the wide open and was nearly pulverized to dust in the disaster. As much as they'd suffered and as peaceful as we tried to prove ourselves, they were too proud and too distrusting of us to let us help them with anything during our stay. Their suspicions of us required that we be in their line of sight at all times and although it made me restless and Kiyahe nervous, we respected their demands.

They were especially scrutinizing of us, making us answer a million questions, studying us for over a week and a half, and questioning everything we said. Their chief worked closely with their elders, their leadership more along the lines of a committee. At first, they did not want to see our letters from other tribes, but when they changed their minds, they poured over the letters, trying to discern whether they were authentic or not. Their history, both with whites and other Natives, didn't help matters. Kiyahe told me that they were forced from their lands numerous times, by white settlers, French fur traders, the Cheyenne, and the Sioux. They were only able to keep their land after they'd fought off smaller tribes and stayed behind while others moved south. Their history and the recent disaster made them especially protective of their lands, which were especially vast compared to the other tribes.

Although we assured them that we were not there to scout and take their land and that we would not let anyone else in our alliance take their land, they were not convinced. It wasn't until I told them that if they did not join our alliance, I couldn't guarantee that others, outside the nation's borders, would not try to conquer them and their lands. Having the numbers, and therefore the support that we'd gained thus far, that is what finally won them over. They joined our united front and wrote and signed another letter of promise. Kiyahe told me that we would especially need their letter when we encountered the Cheyenne and Sioux. I worried that the three tribes wouldn't want to ally with old enemies but Kiyahe assured me that our numbers were large enough that they would rather be with us than against us.

Before we left, the Crow caught me off guard in asking that I sign an agreement of theirs in return. It was written in their Native language and the unfamiliar words made me worry about what they were asking. I felt a wave of sympathy for Natives in the late 1800's who were asked to sign agreements that they could not read. Agreements that they had to trust interpreters to read for them. I was suddenly grateful for Kiyahe and his multi-lingual fluency. He translated it for me and told me that they wanted my promise that their land would not be reduced in any way. The centuries old fear of having their homes taken away was still strong with that tribe. I signed their agreement. Part of me wanted to tell them that, if anything, their lands might expand now that there was so much land unclaimed after the disaster. But I stopped myself, I should not make promises when the future was so vague.

According to Kiyahe's father's map, the Cheyenne had a large reservation in Montana, just east of the Crow reservation. But when we arrived, we found it deserted except for a few hundred skeletons and the charcoaled remains of buildings and vehicles.

We wandered through the ghost town, looking for any sign of survivors and where they might have gone. The four of us spread out in our search, Kiyahe separating from me for the first time since I'd been attacked. The reservation was next to barren and we were always within shouting distance of each other. For once, the wind of the plains was absent, and our voices echoed as we called out to each other across the rubble. At first, I was grateful for the space Kiyahe was giving me, it allowed me to be alone with my thoughts, even for just a little while. But after half an hour or so, the empty houses and silent streets began to feel eerie, the hairs on the back of my neck standing on end and my nervousness growing without my protector by my side.

I was just about to head back to Kiyahe when the screech of a cat caught my attention. I jumped back just as a slender grey cat streaked across the sidewalk in front of me, in hot pursuit of a plump brown mouse. I watched the cat chase the mouse across the dead grass of a lawn and into the open front door of a little blue house.

I stood there looking at the house, mesmerized by it. It was petite, just a hair bigger than a double wide trailer. The siding was painted a robin's egg blue, large strips of paint peeling away from the places where fire had touched. The black shingles on the roof were curling in on themselves, the bricks of the chimney were whitewashed and crumbling. The open front door was made of heavy, sturdy wood and painted a dark navy to match the shutters around the windows. A tricycle and a swing set that was just beginning to rust laid on their sides in the straw-colored grass.

I found myself walking towards the house without consciously deciding to. We had helped repair so many homes in the reservations we'd visited so far. But there was no one to repair this one for. Its owners had either died or abandoned it. In ten years, maybe less, this house would become a ruin just like all the other towns that had been destroyed in the disaster. In the back of my mind I knew it was stupid to pity a house, an inanimate object that had no feelings and knew nothing beyond its own four corners, but I couldn't help myself from feeling sorry for it. For a while, I had known what it was like to be a person without a home. And that home was, and still would be, without an owner.

After righting the tricycle in the front yard, I walked across the threshold and shut the front door behind me. Nearly everything in the house had burnt up. A plush carpet of ash and dust coated the floors and what little furniture was left. My feet stirred up the ashes as I walked, the bottoms of my jeans quickly becoming smudged and stained with the charcoal residue. The kitchen was marked with a mangled sink and battered refrigerator, the bathroom with a quarter of a porcelain toilet still standing, the living room with a half-melted TV set. I had to assume that the last two rooms were bedrooms. The smell of smoke and death rekindled itself without the breeze to blow it away. I had to be careful where I stepped, four corpses littered the various rooms, two adults and two children. The family didn't even have time to find each other in the chaos before they were killed.

I ghosted through the graveyard of the house and into a bedroom. That was where I stepped on a tablet, the glass crackling and spider webbing underneath my blackened tennis shoe. I picked it up, careful not to cut my fingers on the tiny shards. The movement awakened the device and a movie started blaring in my hands. I hurriedly found the volume on the side and dimmed the noise. An animated Pocahontas and John Smith danced through the woods across the screen, Pocahontas singing to her lover about the colors of the wind. I watched the children's movie in my hands with new eyes and understood the lyrics in a way I never had before.

I didn't realize I was crying until my tears plinked onto the cracked screen. And I didn't realize Kiyahe had come into the house, into the room behind me until he laid his hand gently on my shoulder. We watched and listened to the song, which ended just as the battery on the tablet died out. The timing was perfect.

"Ironic, isn't it?" I whispered to Kiyahe in the once again silent house. "They wanted the same thing we want."

Kiyahe pulled me to him then, and we stood there hugging in the remnants of a child's bedroom. Thinking about the past, thinking about the future.

When we caught up with the twins, Neka announced that he'd found hoof prints heading south out of the reservation.

"I'm not sure that really means anything, Neka," Kiyahe shook his head. "An entire herd of horses could have passed through here; it doesn't mean they left on horseback. Besides, their original lands are in the Great Lakes area, it would make more sense for them to head strait east and go there."

"We go to Nebraska next though, right?" I asked. "To the Pawnee?"

"Yes," Kiyahe answered, his eyebrows knitted together in concentration.

"Well let's just make a wide sweep through Wyoming on the way to Nebraska. Maybe we'll find them still travelling like we did with the Navajo. And if there's no sign of them, we hope they'll be in the Great Lakes area and we'll catch them there," I suggested.

Kiyahe mulled it over while I tapped my foot, impatient to get moving considering that they already had a huge head start on us.

"Ok, we'll do a sweep through Wyoming, I can think of a couple places they might be that aren't too far out of our way. Neka, you drive, we need to make this a quick detour."

Neka smirked at his brother, enjoying Kiyahe's agreement that he was the faster driver. Shilah rolled his eyes and the four of us got back on the road.

A day and a half later, we found the Cheyenne and their large herd of horses on their new reservation, just north of the old capital of Cheyenne, Wyoming ironically enough. Like most tribes, they were suspicious of us at first. But once we'd told them how many tribes had joined our alliance and showed them our letters of promise, they joined our cause as well.

From beginning to end, we would visit seventeen tribes on our journey. Those seventeen were the biggest and most renowned. But Ahote had told us before we left that there could be many more out there than what we would encounter. Hundreds more. He believed that the smaller ones would either form their own small communities, travel and join up with larger tribes, or have died out entirely during the Fire Rains. From what we had seen thus far, I guessed that most had either died out or joined larger tribes. I couldn't be sure though; our travels were constricted to where the bus could go and where Kiyahe directed us according to his father's map. I also had to consider the idea that tribes could be travelling to old homelands or new areas altogether, like the Navajo and Cheyenne. We could be missing opportunities to cross paths with tribes by miles.

This was one argument Kiyahe and I always got into, I wanted to search harder for the smaller tribes and try to win them over. I didn't feel content with only winning over seventeen out of hundreds. Kiyahe reminded me that we needed to unite the biggest tribes first because they would be the bulk of our numbers. And he assured me that there would be time to find and meet all the other tribes after we'd returned home and formed something of a new nation. I didn't like it, but I had to admit he was right.

Ahote had also told us that it was very possible we would encounter stragglers, small groups or individuals whose tribes hadn't survived the disaster intact. After over a month and a half of meeting with large tribes, I had all but forgotten that we could run into stragglers. That was until we almost *literally* ran into one.

"What the hell are you doing lady?!" Neka shouted at the windshield as the brakes of the bus screeched and the smell of burning rubber diffused around us. "Get off the damn road you crazy old bat!"

Kiyahe, Shilah, and I darted to the front of the bus to see what Neka was shouting about. Through the dusty windshield, standing in the middle of the highway, was a haggard looking Native woman staring up at our dirty bus.

"I'm gonna give her a piece of my mind," Neka muttered as he threw the gear shift into park and yanked the keys from the ignition. We flew out the door after him.

"Just what the hell do you think you're doing walking in the middle of the damn highway?!" Neka shouted at the woman. The boys held him back as the woman stared between us and the bus with wide eyes. One of her feet stood its ground while the other was turned to run.

"Well there's not exactly a sidewalk out here is there?" the woman said to Neka. She intended the comment to be snarky, but she was too shocked to put the right amount of venom into her response. We all took in a breath after hearing her speak, she looked old enough to be forty, but her voice revealed she couldn't be much older than me. I was the first to recover, knowing what extended travel in the outdoors can make you look like. Can make you *feel* like.

"I'm sorry about my friend, he's a maniac of a driver," I told her. Neka shot me a look of fury but I matched his gaze with a warning in my eyes. He huffed and retreated back into the bus.

"I'm Kaya by the way," I told her. "And this is Kiyahe and Shilah."

"Sorry about my brother, he's an ass," Shilah smiled.

"I'm Dyani, thanks for not running me over," the woman said. She turned her back on us then and walked away.

"Wait!" I yelled, running after her, Kiyahe trailing behind me. "Where are you from?" I asked.

"No where," she answered.

"Where are you going?"

"No where."

"Well we're heading to the Pawnee reservation in Nebraska, do you want a ride?" I tried.

Dyani stopped walking and turned to me then. "No, I don't want a ride, please stop following me."

"Hey," I grabbed her gently by the shoulder and held her until she finally turned her wild eyes to me. "I walked from South Dakota to Oklahoma after the disaster, it's not safe for a woman to be out here alone." I told her. I didn't mention that I hadn't seen a single soul on my journey or that I'd had a protector during that time.

She looked into my eyes for a minute before sighing. "I know, but I'm not going the same direction as you. I'm headed to Kansas to the Kansa reservation."

"Is that where you're from?" I asked her.

"No, I'm from Wyoming," she answered.

I stared at her until finally she blew out a breath and told me her story.

"I'm Teton, from up in Northeast Wyoming. My...my tribe was killed in the disaster," she blinked rapidly and cleared her throat. "I'm the only one left."

I pulled her dirty, grimy self to me then. Her sadness was palpable, and her story was my story. I was the last of my people, too. She let me hold her until she got her emotions under control again. "Anyway," she sniffed. "My aunt married a Kansa man and I'm hoping to find them there."

"We'll take you," I blurted. But then Kiyahe interjected. "It's too far out of the way, Marie. We don't have time," he said softly.

Dyani shook her head then, "You have your path and I have mine. It was nice meeting you though, Marie...or Kaya... what'd you say your name was again?" Dyani wrinkled her eyes in confusion. I had introduced myself as Kaya but Kiyahe had called me Marie. The mix up gave me an idea then.

"It's Kaya," I told her. "And Marie. It's kind of a complicated story, but I'll tell you if you have a minute."

༝

After I'd told Dyani my story and about our journey, she took a minute to think about it. We offered to show her our letters from tribal leaders, but she didn't want them. She said she could see the truth in my eyes.

She promised me her support and Kiyahe had the idea to have her write and sign a letter saying the Teton tribe also supported Kaya. It wasn't a lie; she technically *was* the Teton tribe now. And a letter of yet another tribe's support would further help our cause.

Dyani laughed, "It never occurred to me I could promote myself to chief."

She wrote and signed a quick letter and promised to spread the word of Kaya to anyone she encountered. Even though she was no more than a drop in the ocean, it made me feel good to have taken the time to reach out to her.

We parted ways then, Dyani in search of a new home and family, us in search of a new alliance.

The elders say, 'The longest road you're going to have to walk is from here to here. From your head to your heart.' But they also say you can't speak to the people as a leader unless you've made the return journey. From the heart back to the head.
—Phil Lane, Jr., Yankton Sioux.

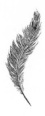

Chapter Nine

A strong wave of nostalgia hit me when we crossed over into Nebraska. With the side of my face pressed against the cold glass of the window by the booth, I wondered if those were the very fields and trees I had walked past just a few months ago. Before I'd found the Potawatomi. Before I'd found my new home and family. Before I'd become Kaya.

That area was also where I'd ran into the wolf, my temporary guardian and protector. It had been a good while since I'd heard his howl and even longer since I'd seen his aquamarine eyes surrounded by snow white fur. After hearing the legend from the Potawatomi, I learned that it wasn't just coincidence that I had run into the gentle giant. He was a part of the plan, the prophecy. It was his job to get me safely to Oklahoma so I could embrace my purpose. Although I would never have traded my new family and purpose for anything, I felt a pinch of jealousy towards the wolf. He had fulfilled his purpose and was now free to roam this new world. I was not. I was bound to my purpose for the rest of my life, until I took my last breath.

When we found the Pawnee, we learned that they had left Oklahoma shortly after the disaster to reclaim their homelands. The men had come first, building homes and preparing the area so that it would be ready for the women, elders, and children when they came.

In talking to them, I learned that I had missed the Pawnee by less than five miles when I'd first passed through.

We got to know the Pawnee as we helped them build homes, wells, and corrals for cattle. The young men and boys were having a blast living like old west cowboys, riding their horses out day after day, roping up lost cattle. The older men worked on tractors, getting them running again so that they would be ready to till and plant come spring time. The women were making clothes, curing meat, and canning goods to stock up for winter. The tribe fell into life on the plains as if they'd never left it. And while we were there, surrounded by flat fields under a vast sky, I suppose we felt like pioneers ourselves.

After a few days of consideration, the Pawnee joined our alliance as well.

The more time I spent with the tribes and their people, the more stories I heard, and the more hours I spent working hard alongside them, the harder it became each time to say goodbye.

But bid them goodbye we did and in the blink of an eye, we were headed north to South Dakota and the Sioux tribe. We would pass directly through my hometown of Atlantis before reaching the reservation.

At first, I didn't want to see my hometown, I wanted Neka to drive the bus around it, out of the way to avoid it. I had tried very hard not to think of my parents and my home since the day I had left it. I was afraid it would re-open the deep gash in my heart and I didn't want the boys to see just how painful the memory was to me. But when we came to the intersection, to the road that would take us around my hometown, it was completely uprooted from the dirt. We had no choice but to go through Atlantis.

"It might not be so bad, Marie. You might be surprised at how well you do. Just try to think of the happy memories, it might even be good for you," Kiyahe had tried to comfort me.

When we first hit the edge of town, I really didn't feel any different. It looked like any other ruin of a town. But then I saw the remnants of the grocery store, the same grocery store I had worked in for two and a half years, the same store I had been in on the day it happened. Suddenly it was hard to breathe, and my eyes pricked with the threat of tears. To make matters worse, Neka had to drive slowly because the roads were so damaged that they were nearly impassable. I closed my eyes and concentrated on each breath until we passed Julio's Supermarket.

I couldn't even remember his laugh or exactly what he looked like anymore.

Kiyahe kept his hand on my shoulder in comfort as we drove through the remains of my hometown. Shilah, seeing my struggle to keep it together, started asking me trivial questions about the town.

"How many people lived here?"

"Where did you go for fun?"

"Did you go to any parties?"

"Were there any cute girls?"

Shilah fired the questions one right after the other so that I didn't have time to get emotional over the topics or the answers, which I guessed was why he did it. He kept my mind moving and I didn't mind playing tour guide for a while.

Atlantis was still a pile of recognizable rubble, but a few things had changed. In the last few months all the corpses had decayed to skeletons, all the smoldering fires had suffocated themselves, all the lighter debris blown away, and all the surrounding grass, vines, and trees had started encroaching. Nature was drowning the ruins, drowning the sadness in greenery. That greenery would brown and die in a month's time, maybe just a few weeks even. Then everything would be covered in a quiet blanket of snow. And when spring returned, the foliage would pick up where it left off, erasing my little community. I wasn't sure whether it would be easier for me when the ruins were gone, or if it would only make the memory hurt more. If I got any say in the matter, I would never return here to find out.

My house used to be on the west side of town, which meant we could stay on the road heading straight north and I wouldn't have to see it if I didn't want to. But then a feeling of cowardice gripped my stomach and I knew that as long as I was here, hopefully for a final time, I should say a proper goodbye to my old life.

"Turn left up here," I directed to Neka. He did as I asked while Kiyahe and Shilah watched me with pity and concern. I stared studiously out the window, avoiding their stares.

When we reached my street, I asked Neka to stop the bus, my voice sounding just as dead as I felt. We stopped, and all three guys followed me as I got out and walked down the street. Less than a block later, on my left was the crater where my house used to be, on my right was the neighbor's house, my refuge during the disaster.

To my left was where my old life ended. To my right was where my new life began.

In a deadpan voice, I told the boys about my parents and the day of the disaster. How I had left the house in an annoyed hurry, how I didn't tell my dad goodbye at all and how I had barely told my mom goodbye. How I didn't tell either of them that I loved them. How I got in my car wishing I was already out of the house and out of town, on my way to college and a new life. How I came back to find a crater, with not even my parents bodies to bury. How I bunkered down in the neighbor's house and forced myself to survive even though I didn't want to. How I felt when I first had the dream that started me on my path.

They listened in silence, I had never told them all this, not even Kiyahe. We had heard so many stories from Natives about the tragedies they'd suffered. Maybe that was another reason I felt so connected to them. Not just because of the legend and my part in it, but because we all knew what it was to lose the things and the people that mattered most. We knew pain, loss, and love.

But most of all, we knew survival, determination, and purpose.

I smiled a small, sad smile, "Mom, dad; I'd like you to meet my protectors and my friends." If the boys thought I was crazy for talking to an empty hole in the ground, they didn't show it. Kiyahe put his hand on my shoulder again.

And then Shilah, God bless him, said, "Hey Kaya's parents! We'll take good care of her for you, I promise!"

The four of us laughed at that and the gloom in the air lifted just a tiny bit.

The twins and I turned to head back to the bus but Kiyahe kept staring solemnly at the crater, his shoes cemented to the ground. I tugged at his arm and he put a steady hand over mine. "I need to tell them something first," he said softly. My eyes glanced up at the twins who were several paces ahead of us now, thinking Kiyahe was talking about them, but Kiyahe continued staring at the place where my parents had died. And then he took a step away from me and towards the edge of the crater.

"I just want to thank you for bringing Marie into this world. I know that were it not for your deaths I would have never met her, and our people would never have known her. And although I don't regret her being here with us, I would trade it all to bring you back for her, to fill the hole in her heart and make her happy again. We *will* take care of her, and I *will* protect her. I promise."

I stared at the planes of his beautiful face, so full of sincerity as he spoke. A part of me was afraid. Before, when he had wanted to keep me from returning to the Apache and other hostile tribes, he had hinted, and once accidentally admitted, that he would trade everything, even the fate of his people, to protect me. And now he was admitting it out loud with no hesitation. This was what his parents had warned about.

But a bigger part of me couldn't help the warmth that was spreading outwards from my core. He just wanted me happy and safe. And the warmth turned into relief when I realized I was overreacting. There was nothing Kiyahe could do to undo the past. We were here, and we had purpose. And it was time to continue the job we had started.

I tugged on Kiyahe's strong arm one more time and he sighed and turned to meet my gaze. His tranquil eyes met my stormy eyes and they communicated all the words that needed saying. Wordlessly, we turned and headed back to the bus.

Kiyahe was right, it hadn't been so bad, and I felt a little bit better.

I even smiled as we drove out of Atlantis.

ↄ⟩

We parked the bus at an RV camp in the heavily wooded area just south of the Sioux reservation. Kiyahe went about his usual scouting while the twins and I set up camp.

That night before we were to meet the largest tribe we had encountered thus far, I had a terrible nightmare.

It started off with another memory, one where I had gone hiking in the woods with my elementary class on a field trip. At the end of the hike would be an open meadow where we would sit and listen to a game and parks officer tell us about all the plants and animals in the area. And then we would have our end of the school year picnic in the sunshine and soft grass. Along the hike, I was carrying a stick that was taller than I was and whapping in on trees and rocks as we walked. It was my weapon in case a bear or a mountain lion tried to eat us. Or so I told myself.

As I walked along, the air grew colder with the chill of autumn and I grew taller with age. The stick was no longer taller than me, in fact it only came up to my ribs after fifty yards or so. When I noticed Kiyahe walking with me on my right, I threw the stick aside. I didn't need it when I had my protector with me.

We walked wordlessly for a while. Until we were down in a valley area of the path, hillsides behind and in front of us. All of a sudden, Kiyahe grabbed my arm and halted both of us.

"What's wrong?" I asked him.

He said nothing as he whipped his head around in all directions, looking and listening for something I could not sense. The trees were dense, and I could see nothing but shadows between them. Then I felt the hairs on my arms and the back of my neck raise, I felt a chill that was not from the crisp breeze. Somehow I knew, and Kiyahe knew, we were being watched. We were being followed.

That was when Kiyahe screamed out in pain, his face pinching and twisting with agony. The sound flushed a flock of birds out of the trees above us and shattered the silence of the forest.

The forest went black around me before I could figure out what had happened.

Of course, I was overly cautious and anxious the next morning.

The more I kept having these premonition-like dreams, the more I started to believe that what the Hopi chief's wife had assumed about me was true.

That I was a shaman.

What that meant for me as Kaya and what that meant for the Potawatomi, I had no idea. And I was too afraid to suggest the idea to Kiyahe.

So instead of worrying about the future, I worried about our present objective: meeting the Sioux. I knew nothing about the tribe that was located less than thirty miles from my hometown of Atlantis. But Kiyahe had said it would be our biggest alliance yet and that the Sioux's history was one of violent conquest. Their numbers had made them one of the largest tribes of their time and they had fought over and won a significant amount of land from their smaller neighbors and enemies. The whites had promised them that they could keep their sacred lands until it was discovered that there was gold underneath them. They battled with stubborn determination until they were eventually forced out of the area.

"It won't be easy to convince them to join an alliance when they have the numbers and land that they have," Kiyahe had warned Shilah and I as he cleaned his grandfather's pistol at the booth. "They don't need the help or the protection that the smaller tribes do."

"So basically, it'll be like trying to convince the biggest kid on the playground to share his toys," Neka confirmed, pessimism filling his voice as he sighed heavily.

"Hey if a pretty girl like Kaya asked you to share your toys, I bet you would," Shilah said, giving me a wink.

"I'd share a lot more than just my toys…" Neka said slyly, waggling his eyebrows.

My face flamed with embarrassment as the twins laughed at my expense. When they noticed Kiyahe's warning look they coughed to hide their chuckles and averted their eyes to the floor.

I brought the attention back to the day's work then. "If they lost so much, I'd think they'd be fired up more than anyone else to prevent it from happening again," I thought aloud.

Kiyahe smiled at me with pride. "Maybe that's how you can put it to them to make them listen."

Kiyahe's rare and beautiful smiles always ignited a flurry of feelings in me. My immediate response was always to smile back, as if reflecting his happiness would make it stay on his face even longer. On the outside I felt hot, like I was melting. In my stomach I felt fluttery, in my head I felt dizzy, and in my heart I felt warm and peaceful. In the five seconds that his smile lingered, I forgot all about my duty and my worries.

The twins, of course, could always be counted upon to snap me out of it. Kiyahe went to the cupboard where we kept the weapons and ammunition and, while his back was turned, the twins looked between Kiyahe and I, waggled their eyebrows, and dramatically feinted like lovesick ladies. My blush returned with full force and I turned my face from their snickering to the window, letting my hair cover up the flush of heat on my neck and face.

Neka stayed behind with the bus as Kiyahe, Shilah, and I walked into the depths of the forest, towards the Sioux reservation. As soon as we were surrounded by dense pines, shrubbery, and shadows, I stuck behind Kiyahe so tightly that we could have been conjoined twins. The forest wasn't like the ones around Atlantis or the ones surrounding the Spokane reservation. It was dark, dense, and eerie. The hairs on the back of my neck and along my arms stood on end, goosebumps making little hills between the straight strands. I glanced to Shilah at my side, his charcoal eyes darted everywhere, and I could sense he was just as nervous as I was. If something or someone came at us, we wouldn't see them until they were toe-to-toe with us.

I felt the chill as we entered the valley. I stopped in the middle of it, one hill behind us, one in front. Shilah stopped with me right away but Kiyahe took several more steps before realizing we weren't with him. He returned to me instantly, his face a mirror of my own fear.

"What's wrong?" he asked me.

"I don't…this is…no, no, no, no!" I started to panic, my eyes flying across the trees too fast to see. My breathing raced on the verge of hyperventilation and my heart pounded with the fury of a locomotive. It was coming, what exactly I didn't know but I could *feel* it!

"Marie! What's wrong?!" Kiyahe shouted at me, shaking my shoulders with his strong hands. My eyes flitted across Shilah, who was searching the trees, trying to find whatever it was I was looking for.

"Kiyahe you have to go! It's going to hurt!" I shouted at him.

"What's going to hurt?!" he shouted back, my panic fueling his.

And as soon as the words were out, he screamed, his face twisting in agony just like it had in my nightmare. The birds screamed with him as they flew out of the tops of the trees in large flocks. His fingers dug into the tops of my shoulders just as mine gripped his tense biceps. I fell with him onto the dirt floor of the forest, only faintly hearing the sound of yips and shouts from men, hidden in the shadows.

Kiyahe lurched himself up from his back to look at the arrow that had pierced his calf. The arrow had sunk itself clear through his leg and blood was seeping out around the shaft on either side. He gritted his teeth as he tried to get up, I guessed to fire back at whoever had shot him. My eyes were glued to the wound as he moved, blood flowing out like a steady stream.

My survival instincts from my days journeying across the plains kicked in and I gently shoved him back down. He tried to sit back up, refusing to be still.

"Stop it! Movement makes the bleeding worse," I commanded. I was kneeling in the dirt with Kiyahe's head resting on my thigh. Quickly, I shrugged out of my jacket and ripped long strips from the bottom of my cotton long sleeve shirt, tying them around the shaft of the arrow beside the entrance and exit wounds. As I bandaged Kiyahe and reduced my shirt to a crop top, Shilah pointed his loaded gun at the eight Sioux men who had us surrounded. The men aimed right back at the three of us with guns and arrows, a standoff forming.

A man moved towards Kiyahe and in the blink of an eye I ripped Kiyahe's grandfather's pistol from the holster at his side and aimed it right between the man's eyes. He jumped back and raised his hands in surrender. I'd never fired a pistol before, but I tried to hold it like I knew exactly what I was doing. If I hadn't had a wounded protector in my lap, I would have gone for my own weapon.

The thought of my bow drew my eyes to the bow slung across the man's bare chest, and I realized he was probably the one who had shot my protector. I returned my blazing eyes to the man's face. He wore an amused, almost taunting expression.

"I just wanted my arrow back," the man smiled slyly.

"Come and get it," I dared him. He smiled wider, clearly enjoying himself.

"What's your business here?" A male voice from the left side of the circle demanded. I hoped Shilah had the male voice in his crosshairs because I was not taking my eyes off the man in front of me.

"We come to see your chief," I answered loudly and clearly without taking my eyes off the man armed with the bow in front of me. He had the nerve to wink at me and I pulled the hammer back, the click catching everyone's attention and wiping the smirk off the bow man's face.

"What do you need to see the chief for?" the other man continued, ignoring my twitchy trigger finger. It was less that I really wanted to shoot the bow man and more that I was shaking in my boots because I was so nervous.

"It's for the chief's ears only. If he decides to tell you that's his business," I answered.

Instead of arguing like I thought the voice would, he fell silent in consideration. And then he decided, "Bring them. Help the wounded one."

Thankfully, two different men came to help Kiyahe out of my arms while the bow man walked beside me, his stupid grin returning. Shilah stuck close behind me and I followed, inches behind Kiyahe and the men helping him walk.

Just a quarter mile north, we started a climb up the grassy side of a cliff. At the top, I could see the smoke from several fires. It's a defense tactic, I realized. They could see all from above and outsiders could only reach them from one side of the cliff. They were very smart, as Kiyahe had predicted.

The thought of my protector drew my eyes back to him. Kiyahe was gritting his teeth but couldn't help the occasional moan of pain that slipped between his lips as he struggled uphill. I fought the urge to reach out to him and tried to keep my face brave and placid.

I wasn't sure if the nightmare was over or just beginning.

But above all, you should understand that there can never be peace between nations until it is known that true peace is within the souls of men.

–Black Elk, Oglala Lakota Sioux.

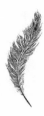

Chapter Ten

The man who had brought us to the tribe, we learned, was the chief's nephew and next in line to become chief.

Kiyahe was taken to the healer so that he could be tended to. I started to throw a fit, remembering what had happened the last time we were separated, but Kiyahe, gritting his teeth through the pain, promised me he would be alright and before I could argue further, Kiyahe was helped into the healer's tipi and the chief's nephew was escorting Shilah and I to the chief's home.

The chief and shaman, a husband and wife both in their mid-fifties, were cold and unfriendly towards us. When I learned of their misfortunes though, I couldn't say I blamed them. They had lost their oldest child, a son, in the disaster, and their second child, a daughter, was about my age and was sick with some sort of stomach problem. The name of the diagnosis was so long that I couldn't pronounce it, yet alone remember it. She had been getting professional medical treatment until the local hospital was blown to pieces in the disaster. Since there were no more hospitals, doctors, or even electricity for that matter, their daughter had nowhere to go to receive treatment. Without science and the advanced world we used to live in, they were reduced to relying on the tribe's healer to help their last living child. And from the look of her, it didn't appear she would survive much longer. They had chosen their nephew, the son of the chief's sister, to become the next chief in preparation for their daughter's demise.

I could see the disaster, the Fire Rains, in their sunken eyes and knew that they would not look back on the disaster as a new chapter or a chance to start over. They would look back on that day as the day that their children were taken from them.

I wanted to tell them about my own losses, but I didn't because just by looking at them, I knew they wouldn't be able to hear me through their own pain.

Before we could launch into our story, the chief sent his nephew to go get his sister, the chief's niece, and bring her so that she could listen as well. It was already overly crowded in the chief's quaint cabin home with not even enough chairs for the six of us, but I didn't complain. They were giving me a chance to speak without any trouble or complaint and for that I was grateful. When the chief's niece arrived, she glared at me in anger. I would have thought the glaring was because of my skin color, or because of my intrusion on her tribe and her family. But then I saw that she shared her look of irritation with everyone and about everything. And I would soon learn that it wasn't just a look she wore, but a dominant part of her personality. And it would be not long after that that I learned *why* she was so full of bitterness. For that moment though, I tried not to take it personally as I launched into my story.

I finished and there were a few moments of silence before the chief's niece asked to be excused. Her words dripped with disdain and she left before anyone could give her an answer. No one chased after her or commented on her rudeness. I realized then that she was included out of some old-fashioned ritual of family tradition and not because anyone really cared about her opinion.

And then the chief commanded my attention with the words he spoke between gritted teeth. "I bury my son in the ground with my own two hands and watch my daughter waste away by the hour and you still ask this of me?"

I flinched at the ice in the chief's voice and the way he talked of his daughter's imminent death like she wasn't even in the room. I looked to his wife and daughter then, who stared at the ground with exhaustion and grief.

"I wasn't exactly ready for this either," I answered him. "I lost both of my parents in the disaster, my whole family. And after a month of surviving alone I found out this is what I've been spared for. I'm still grieving, just as you are."

The chief's nostrils flared at my words. His mourning had been interrupted by my arrival. But I couldn't help it, I had a responsibility not just to my own tribe, but to his and all the others as well. Maybe it was a lapse in patience or maybe it was my fear of how Kiyahe was doing, but my next words were sharper than before.

"We are picking ourselves up and dusting ourselves off just like every other nation. And the longer we sit here, the more organized everyone else becomes. We need to stand united with the other tribes and declare this land as our own. And we need to continue protecting that claim so that history doesn't repeat itself," I told him, trying to sound as strong and determined as possible without sounding demanding and patronizing.

The chief looked at his gathered family then and I guessed that he was considering his ancestors pain and whether or not he was at risk for putting his own family through that pain. The pain of being conquered and reduced to almost nothing.

"I need more time," he finally said in a soft voice. I wondered if he meant more time to consider or more time to grieve. "Go back to your camp and we will talk more tomorrow."

My stomach dropped then, "I can't leave my protector here alone." I tried not to let the fear into my voice, but my attempt was futile.

"You have my promise he will not be harmed, he will be fine with the healer," the chief said.

"I…can't," I stammered. When the chief looked at me, anger returning to his features I explained. "*I* can't leave *him*," I admitted. And it was true, I wasn't trying to be a nuisance. Kiyahe was my weakness and every minute we spent separated made me nervous.

"They can stay with Aiyana," the chief's wife piped in then. "It's the least our niece could do after leaving so rudely."

The chief acquiesced, and his nephew took us to his sister's tipi. She threw us a look of contempt from the cot that she laid on when we walked in but didn't say anything. As her brother explained that we would be staying with her as guests until Kiyahe was healed, she looked at the posts sticking up out of the tipi, completely bored.

Her brother left, and so did Shilah after we agreed that Neka needed to know of our spending the night so he wouldn't be worried. Shilah was uncomfortable leaving me without a protector, but I assured him I would be alright. Aiyana wasn't friendly, but she didn't appear violent. Just bored and annoyed. Shilah left me his pistol and ducked out, promising to check on Kiyahe on his way back. It was just us girls then.

The silence was deafening but when I opened my mouth to start small talk, nothing came out. I perched on the edge of another cot on the far side of the tipi from Aiyana and silently prayed that Kiyahe would be alright while I stared at the dirt floor.

"Would you stop fidgeting, already? Your boyfriend's gonna be fine," Aiyana rolled her eyes at me.

I didn't realize I had been shifting restlessly and picking at my finger nails until Aiyana's icy voice cut through my thoughts.

"I'm sorry, I…" but she turned her attention back to the tipi posts. Then, after two seconds of quiet I muttered, "and he's not my boyfriend."

Aiyana snorted, unconvinced and I decided to ignore her. I laid down on my cot, letting my spine and muscles unkink and unwind. The stress of this trip, the constant travelling, and the emotional rollercoasters were prematurely aging me. I felt like an eighty-five-year-old woman who had walked the length of the world and experienced everything in it.

"You can try to convince my uncle til you're blue in the face, but it won't work," Aiyana said then.

"What do you mean?" I asked.

"I mean he doesn't care about your prophecy or the future. He only cares about his dying daughter and already dead son. He doesn't see anything else."

I was surprised at the callous tone she used when talking about her dead and dying cousins. I opened my mouth to respond but then shut it again. This girl was convinced I would fail here and I didn't want to talk about or even think about that possibility. This tribe was just as important to ally with as all the others. Instead I changed the subject.

"So, where's your parents? I didn't see them back at the chief's house."

I immediately regretted the new topic. Aiyana flinched at the word 'parents,' my question striking a nerve. But she was tougher than me. The pinched look of pain was covered up almost as quickly as it was revealed.

"My dad took off when I was three and I haven't seen him since. My mom's across the way, staying with some other patients."

"Patients?" She flinched again but I couldn't keep the question from spilling out.

"She's a severe paranoid schizophrenic and she hallucinates. She and the other two patients were in an asylum before it got blown to bits," Aiyana said matter of factly.

I had nothing to say to that. I could've said sorry again, but I got the feeling she didn't want to hear my apology. It wouldn't make anything any better.

Thankfully, Shilah came back only thirty minutes or so after he'd left and said Kiyahe was doing fine. The healer had broken both ends of the arrow off and removed the shaft from his leg. Then he had cleaned and cauterized both ends of the wound, bandaged his leg, and gave him pain pills and medicine to help him sleep. The process sounded brutal to me and I wished I had been there to help him through it, but it was too late then.

"Can I go see him?" I asked Shilah, as if he was the healer.

"I don't see why they wouldn't let you, but he's drugged up and sleeping so you won't be able to talk to him," he shrugged.

I caught sight of Aiyana rolling her eyes at me just before I darted out of the tipi.

Kiyahe was, as Shilah had said, sleeping. I crouched next to the low gurney with mangled legs that the healer was using as a hospital bed. Kiyahe was covered in a sheen of sweat on his face and bare torso, but he seemed peaceful and pain-free in his sleep. The healer, a burly and brutish man, harrumphed when I'd demanded to see him.

"He's not dying girl, he's young and strong and he'll be fine," the man had growled at me. But he stood aside and let me see him all the same.

A couple minutes later, the healer left to take some brewed concoction that smelled like cabbage and armpit to the chief's daughter. Her 'stomach medicine,' as he'd called it. I wasn't a doctor, so I couldn't know whether the brew was helping the emaciated, hollow girl I'd seen earlier, but it sure as hell smelled like a miserable treatment.

I shifted so that I was kneeling and watched Kiyahe sleep awhile. I found a fairly clean rag on a rickety, handmade bedside table and wiped his sweat away. Then I traced the planes of his face and torso with my finger. I knew I shouldn't, but the feel of his smooth, warm skin underneath my finger felt nice and brought me a sense of peace. After tracing him a third time, I gently, ever so gently, laid my head on his chest. I closed my eyes and listened to his heartbeat pulse beneath my ear. I breathed in the fresh linen scent of him.

Seventy-two heartbeats later, I lifted my head and kissed the strong jaw of his face. I was crossing the line of where our relationship was supposed to be. And even if he wasn't conscious to know it, I would still feel the guilt later.

But for the moment, the warmth inside me felt so good that I didn't care what pain or guilt the actions brought me. If that was as close as I would ever get to being with Kiyahe in the way my heart compelled me to, then I would remember and treasure those moments always.

ॐ

That night I had a dream that my grandparents were taking me to the hospital to see my new baby cousin. I was little, four or five at the most, and I held on to both of their hands as we crossed the hot summer parking lot in front of the newly remodeled hospital. My parents were coming to visit later, they were watching my other cousins and taking care of my aunt and uncle's house while they were away. I bounced impatiently as my grandma spoke with the receptionist, and giggled happily when they let me push the buttons for the elevator.

The long hallway of the maternity ward stretched out in front of us. As we walked along, it only got longer. And I only got bigger, older. When I looked to my right, my grandpa was gone, and I was holding the hand of the Sioux chief. To my left, in place of my grandma, was the chief's wife. They looked worse than I remembered. As if *they* were the ones who were sick and not their daughter.

When we got to the correct room, I knew I would see the Sioux chief's daughter and not my baby cousin. As I opened the door and stepped in, I grimaced in preparation for what I would see.

Just as I crossed the threshold, a bright light blinded me.

When I blinked my vision clear, I was no longer in the hospital with the Sioux chief and his wife. I was in a grassy field and it was spring time. The sun shone brightly, and I lifted my hand to shield my eyes from its glare. Fifty yards or so away from me, in a field of little green clovers, was a young Native man. From a distance it appeared that his face had been badly burned as it was marred with ugly pink and white scars. He beckoned be forward and I walked closer to him, curious.

When I reached him, the scars had disappeared and he was handsome and glowing. He looked familiar, his features reminded me of the Sioux chief's daughter, but I couldn't place where I'd seen him before. He smiled at me with pearly teeth and took my hand. Before I could protest or pull back, he'd gently pried open my fisted left hand and put what looked like a clover in my palm. I looked at the clover for a minute, unsure of what the hell I was supposed to do with it. I raised my eyes to look at him and opened my mouth to thank him.

But he was gone. I looked all around me, but he was nowhere to be seen. It was just me, standing in a patch of clovers. Strangely, the dream hadn't ended. So not knowing what else to do, I sat and picked clovers while I waited for him to come back. Or for the dream to be over, whichever came first. I had a lapful of the little green flora when I heard a howl and the blinding light returned.

I was back in the hospital, staring at an empty hospital bed. Well, it was empty of a patient anyways. My lapful of clovers was in a pile on the bed. I heard the wolf's howl one more time before I was pulled from the dream back to the cozy room of Aiyana's tipi.

جرح

While Aiyana and Shilah slept, I laid there waiting for dawn, trying to understand yet another strange dream.

Slowly, I had begun to come to terms with the Hopi shaman's conclusion that I was a shaman myself. But I hadn't told a soul. I was afraid of the complications it would cause. How could I be a leader of all these tribes *and* be the next shaman of the Potawatomi? I couldn't do both jobs!

Could I?

My head swum with the idea of it, the job I had already was so overwhelming. And what kind of shaman would I be anyway? I could never figure out these premonitions, these *visions*, until *after* they had come to fruition. What good did that do me? What good did that do anybody?

Shilah and I spent the next couple days trying to convince the Sioux chief to ally with us. We addressed every angle we could think of, but he just kept saying that he needed more time. Every day his daughter grew paler and weaker than the last. After the third day, he couldn't even take his eyes off her to look at us as we discussed an alliance. She truly *was* dying, and the healer's brews weren't curing her or even easing her symptoms.

After the fifth day, she couldn't leave her bed to be a part of the meetings.

When I'd first arrived that day and didn't see her, I was afraid she had died but her tired mother assured me she was just tired. Her being 'just tired' went on for two more days.

As the chief's daughter got worse, Kiyahe got better. The healer equipped him with crutches and he hobbled around behind us as we met with the chief and his wife and got to know the Sioux people. Aiyana followed along with us, cynical and bored but quiet and tolerable.

One brisk morning we were out with the women, picking berries before they were ruined by the first freezes of the season. We picked all morning and ate lunch down by a small stream. Across the water from us was an open field, one that the Sioux would use next spring for planting crops.

"What grows over there now?" I asked Aiyana before taking a bite of my turkey sandwich.

"Nothing much, just grass and weeds I think," Aiyana shrugged taking a swig of water from her canteen.

"Huh," I muttered, looking across the water at the green field. The short green, leafy stems looked almost like the clovers from my dreams.

"Hey, I'm gonna take a look around over there, I'll be right back," I told Aiyana as stood and wiped my hands on my jeans. She nodded, "I'll go with you," and stood with my protectors to follow me.

The stream was shallow but moving swiftly. I quickly kicked off my hiking boots and peeled off my socks. After I had my jeans rolled up to my knees, I took the first step into the frigid water, gasping at the chill. The three of them followed suit and we waded the ten feet across the racing stream to the field on the other side. I had carried my boots and socks over, but I didn't put them back on, the fielded area was soft underfoot and covered, indeed, with the little green clovers from my dream.

The far-off sound of a wolf echoed in the air.

"Does your healer use these for anything?" I asked Aiyana as I bent down to pluck a clover.

"If it stinks or it tastes bad he probably does," Aiyana sniveled. "He gave my mom some kind of vine to smoke to help calm her when she has a break down, but it didn't work and it took me a week to get the reeking smell out of her clothes." Aiyana couldn't see my face to see me grimace. In the time that we'd spent there, I learned quickly that nobody particularly cared for Aiyana. She was snarky and sarcastic. And she always had someone or something to complain about. She was practically an orphan and her brother and extended family didn't pay much attention to her unless it was to nag at her. Kiyahe and Shilah didn't make a point of talking to her either. I appeared to be the only one who tolerated and included her. In truth, I think it was because I understood her. I understood what it was to lose parents and to feel alone.

We just expressed ourselves differently.

"They don't look like they'd be good for much except for seasoning maybe," Kiyahe observed, pulling my attention back to the field.

I thought back to my dream and wondered… could they be used as medicine? Could they ease or even cure whatever was wrong with the chief's daughter? If we brewed a tea out of them or even fed them to her straight…everyone would think I was insane if I suggested the idea. And even if they tried it, they would be shocked if it worked. I was no doctor or healer.

But I was *probably* a shaman.

And that meant I should heed whatever my dreams were trying to tell me.

"Help me pick these," I told them. "I have something to tell you guys while we pick."

To say everyone was shocked was an understatement.

They were dumbfounded.

Aiyana was the first to recover. "So, let me get this straight; you've had this dream night after night since you've been here, the potential cure to save my cousin's life, and you didn't tell anybody?! Jesus, Kaya, the girl is dying and you kept this to yourself all this time?!"

"I don't know if it's a cure! It could just be a crazy dream, for all I know!" I shouted back at her.

"This isn't some déjà vu bullshit, Kaya! That Hopi woman wasn't pulling ideas out of her ass for your entertainment! You *are* a shaman Kaya and we have to take these weeds to the healer right now!"

"Hold on a second!" Kiyahe intervened. "If these clovers don't work, we don't want to get everyone's hopes up for nothing," Kiyahe rationalized. "I agree we take them to the healer, but we can't go around explaining a hunch as the work of a shaman unless we know *for sure*."

I nodded, in total agreement. There wasn't time to wrap our heads around the idea of me being a shaman, we had to try and save a life first.

"They've got nothing to lose," I said. "If it doesn't work, then we know I'm not a shaman and that it was just a crazy dream, no harm done."

"And if it does work," Aiyana added. "Then you've saved the girl's life, *and* you're a shaman, *and* my uncle owes you the alliance of our tribe."

And with that we gathered up our small harvest and splashed across the stream, back to the reservation to save the chief's daughter and find out once and for all what was behind my foreshadowing dreams.

Where there is vision, the people live. They are made rich in the things of the spirit; and then, as the logical next step, they are rich in human life.

–Phil Lane, Sr., Yankton Sioux.

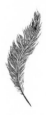

Chapter Eleven

It took a good while to convince the healer to administer the clovers to the chief's daughter. Kiyahe told him he'd seen his grandmother use similar looking clovers to heal ulcers that a man in our tribe had had and thought they might help the chief's daughter with her stomach problems as well. The healer ranted and raved that the clovers were useless and that they might even be poisonous if ingested. The mention of 'poisonous' caught my attention and made me consider. What if these didn't help the chief's daughter at all? What if they even *killed* her?

But then I got that feeling in the pit of my stomach and in the core of my heart that my premonition was right, the clovers would help her. They would save her life. The healer finally acquiesced when we threatened to take the clovers and our idea to the chief and treat her ourselves.

So, the healer made a brewed tea of the tiny stems with little green leaves and the four of us followed him to the chief's home. Kiyahe explained his hunch again and the chief, with the face of a man who was close to losing his sanity, gave his permission for us to give the tea to his daughter. The four of us had decided that if it worked, we would tell the chief the truth about my vision-like dreams and how they'd brought me to the clovers. And if it didn't, Kiyahe would take responsibility and say that it must have been different clovers his grandmother had used.

By the end of the day, the chief's daughter was well enough to leave her bed and eat a full meal.

By the next day, her eyes were less cloudy, and some color was coming back into her face.

And by the next day, she was helping some of the older women do some light work around the reservation.

With Kiyahe, Shilah, and Aiyana beside me as my witnesses, I poured out all I knew about my dreams to the chief, his family, and the healer. The healer stood in the corner of the room with his arms crossed, miffed that I had been the one responsible for curing his dying patient instead of him. All eyes were on the Sioux chief, waiting for his commentary.

"I think we have a shaman, and a very powerful one at that, standing before us. I cannot think of any other way to explain your foreshadowing gifts except that they are a blessing from the Great Spirit. You are truly a blessed child of His. And we would be honored to stand in alliance with you."

I blushed at his observation and approval. The secrecy of my dreams was out now, and word would spread that Kaya's discovered abilities saved a Sioux chief's dying daughter from death. I still didn't know what this would mean for my own tribe or how they'd take the news when we got home, but I hoped everything would turn out alright. Shilah and Neka seemed to think it would.

But Kiyahe hadn't said a word about it since I'd revealed the truth about my dreams in the clover field. He'd been awkwardly avoiding me, as much as a soul-bound protector could anyways, and he never put in his two-cents when the subject was talked about. I didn't push to know what he was thinking, I only hoped he would be ok with it and that his parents would come to the same conclusion when we told them.

We spent Thanksgiving with the Sioux. At first, I thought it a bit odd, celebrating a holiday that had started with the budding relationship between whites and Natives that would, over the course of a couple centuries, turn sour. But the chief and his wife, both looking happier and healthier in parallel to their daughter's improving health, insisted it was absolutely appropriate for the circumstances.

"After all," the smiling Sioux shaman had told me lovingly, "You have saved our daughter from death just as our ancestors saved your ancestors from death. The saving of a life and the alliance we've made is certainly something to be thankful for."

"And I would bet that the other tribes you have visited will be thankful for what you have done as well," the chief added.

I thought back to the tribes we had visited, hoping what the chief said was true. Hoping they were thankful for our new alliances and not regretful. I wondered if the tribes we had yet to meet would celebrate Thanksgiving. I hoped they could find something to be thankful for in the time since the disaster.

The night before our departure, the first snow fell, and the frigid temperatures allowed it to stick and build. There was an indoor celebration in the Sioux lodge and everyone was thrilled with the new alliance and the knowledge that the chief's daughter would live to take her place as a Sioux leader. The chief and his wife drank and laughed with their tribe, happy to be celebrating instead of planning a funeral for their last living child. Aiyana's brother, who would not become chief now that his cousin was in line to take her rightful place as a shaman, quietly accepted the alternative position the chief had bestowed upon him. He was now a tribal elder and although he was decades younger than the other elders, the chief saw it fitting as he'd done so much as chief-to-be and hadn't complained once about his demotion.

After the meal, I stood by Kiyahe and Aiyana by the chief's head table. We watched and laughed at the twins' attempts to charm the Sioux girls. Aiyana excused herself to go to the bathroom just as a slow song was starting up, leaving me and my primary protector alone.

"Will you dance with me?" Kiyahe asked after a moment, his soft tone barely audible over the din of the party. I glanced from the twins to Kiyahe's strong, bronze hand held out to me. I hesitated, remembering the last time we had slow danced and I had run out on him. But then I looked into those tranquil blue eyes and before I could consider the risks, I found myself on the dance floor, letting him lead me.

As the song, "All the Pretty Girls," by Kaleo started, I remembered back to the last time I had slow danced with Kiyahe. The warmth of his hold and the magnetizing draw of his eyes. The way he had tilted his face towards mine. I tried to skip over the part where I had run away from him. At the time, I had thought I was afraid of what people would think, what they would say, how it would affect their view of me as a leader. But now I realized that that wasn't really what I was afraid of.

I was afraid of falling in love.

Kiyahe noticed my grimace at the memory and leaned his head down so that our foreheads were touching, our breath mingling and our faces so close together that my heart stuttered.

"What's wrong, Marie?" he asked, his words coated with concern and his breath warm on my face.

I pulled away slightly so that I could think straight, but the instant our eyes met I found myself pouring out my heart to him. My worry resurfacing about what being a shaman could mean.

"The legend didn't say that Kaya was a shaman, wouldn't that be an important detail? What does it mean? What…how can I be two things at once? Why is all of this being put on my shoulders? What does it mean for…us?" the questions fell out of my mouth, one right after the other before I could give Kiyahe a chance to answer them.

Kiyahe smiled as if my fears were those of a child seeing monsters in the shadows of their bedroom. "The legend didn't say Kaya was a shaman, but it didn't say Kaya *couldn't* be a shaman either. And the Great Spirit wouldn't have given you these responsibilities, these *blessings* if He knew you couldn't handle them. Everything will be ok, Marie."

Kiyahe maneuvered me so that we were dancing in the back of the room in front of a massive blazing fireplace, away from the other dancers. I looked around to see if anyone was watching us, but all the couples seemed only interested in their partners.

"But *why*?" I moaned, "I just don't understand *why*."

"It's all His plan, Marie. It's all for a reason, for a purpose. Sometimes we don't learn the answer until we're face-to-face with Him. At the end."

I chewed my lip while I thought about that. It seemed a very long time to wait.

"But I do have…a theory," Kiyahe hesitated, his eyes looking everywhere but at me, as if he was afraid to admit his thoughts.

"What theory?" I pressed.

He swallowed, "Well…your last question, about what this means for us?" I nodded, a blush spreading across my chest and up my neck.

"I wonder if maybe, the Great Spirit or God or whoever…maybe He *knew*. Maybe He *knows*, that I have feelings for you," Kiyahe whispered. "And that you have feelings for me?" Kiyahe whispered the words as a question. But before I could answer he continued.

"And if He did, if He *does*," Kiyahe said louder. "Then maybe that's how this is supposed to be. I'll be the next chief; you'll be the next shaman. I'll be by your side as your protector for life. And you'll lead the people. We'll be together, fulfilling our part of the plan."

Kiyahe's touch, and the blaze of the fireplace, warmed my outsides but I could feel a growing warmth *inside* me too. One of rightness, one of truth, one of hope and love.

One of happiness.

If being a shaman helped me fulfill the promise I'd made in being Kaya, if it enabled me to be with Kiyahe the way I really wanted to be, I would accept it gladly. A thousand times over.

We smiled at each other, the glow from the fire not nearly as bright as the glow inside of us.

"I want that to be true, I love you," I confessed, and happy tears that had not touched my eyes in a good while flowed steadily then. Consequences and fears be damned.

"I *know* it's true," Kiyahe said. "I may not be a shaman, but I can feel it. And I love you too."

He kissed me then, long and thoroughly. Our mouths weren't quite sure how to move at first, but then that constant spark of electricity and heat ignited, and we kissed like we would never get the chance to do it again. He pulled me to him, his strong arms wrapping around my waist. My arms were just as tight around his neck and my hands tangled in his tousled, raven black hair. The song came to a close as the kiss ended and we smiled at each other without fear or hesitation.

I'd found my home away from home.

After our confessions and that first kiss, we decided that it was best to keep our PDA to a minimum in front of the tribes. Although almost everyone we had come into contact with had probably assumed that Kiyahe and I were together (or if they had predicted that we would be eventually), we still wanted to show that we were focused and determined on our mission.

When we were at the bus though, we let our guards down around the twins. They had known what we had been denying ever since the first night we'd met them. With Kiyahe and I's obvious feelings for each other out in the open, the twins took to teasing us mercilessly.

"You guys aren't gonna fool around in the bedroom now are you? Because if you are, we're tenting it outside," Neka joked.

"Hell no, dude," Shilah shook his head. "It's too damn cold out there."

"Well if you'd stop scaring off the girls we meet maybe I could bring a couple back one of these times to keep us warm," Neka waggled his eyebrows.

"A lot of good that would do you," Shilah retorted. "Girls want a guy with some meat to keep them warm, not a toothpick like you."

"That's not meat, that's cellulite. A.K.A hail damage."

"I'll show you some kind of damage all right!"

Shilah threw himself from one couch across to the other, on top of his brother. A wrestling match ensued before Kiyahe, who was sitting up front examining the map again, scolded them like children and they returned to their respective couches, both of them panting.

"But really Kaya," Shilah said quietly so Kiyahe couldn't hear him. "Do we need to soundproof the walls or are you and Negative Nancy up there gonna contain yourselves?"

"Shut up guys," I rolled my eyes at them, my blush flaming up my throat and face.

"Look how red she's getting bro, could you be any more obvious about being a virgin Kaya? Just write it on your forehead for God's sake," Neka chuckled.

"Do you need a how-to book so you'll know what to do?" Shilah laughed.

"Shut up already, it's none of your business!" I hissed at them.

"Hey, we're your protectors, you *are* our business," Shilah countered.

Neka smiled slyly, "Yeah Kaya, just looking out for you is all."

"Careful Kaya, you blush any deeper and someone really is gonna confuse you with a red skin!" Shilah nearly burst.

"I'll punch those smiles right off your faces!" I yelled. Kiyahe turned around at that.

"Oooh is that a threat or a promise?" Neka winked.

The twins howled with laughter and nearly fell off of their couches in the process. I got up with my fists clenched, ready to throw blows at both of their stupid faces but it only made them laugh harder. I turned around when I heard a third snicker behind me and Kiyahe quickly tried to cover up his smile. I couldn't help but fight a smile myself, seeing his eyes light up and the corners of his mouth twitch.

But then a knock on the bus door silenced everyone and we froze solid in shock, wondering who had found our well-hidden bus, nestled in an abandoned, shady campground a mile southeast of the Sioux reservation. We darted to the windows to see Aiyana standing outside with a sour expression, shivering.

Kiyahe opened the door and the brisk cold followed her entry. She pulled her thin cotton gloves off and blew on her hands to warm them up.

"God, it's freezing out there, did you have to park so far away?" she asked, her voice full of her usual irritation.

"It's a precaution we take every time," Kiyahe said, taking her damp coat from her and hanging it on a nail on the wall.

Aiyana slid into the booth across from me and Kiyahe slid in next to me. I tried to ignore the buzzing electricity that coursed between our touching arms and to focus on Aiyana's face instead. She truly was very pretty once you were able to see past her cloud of petulance. Her dark eyes were infinitely deep, and her skin was smooth and mocha colored. Her black eyebrows arched sharply over her eyes and her hair hung in straight glossy strands around her face and halfway down her back.

"I heard you're leaving," she started.

"Yes, we're going northeast across the Canadian border, to the Blackfoot," I said.

She nodded, "I want to go with you."

The boys all bristled, no one particularly cared for Aiyana and her sulky attitude except for me. I looked between them and could see that they didn't want her to travel with us.

"What about your family? And your tribe?" I asked.

"My family doesn't care, I'm just a nuisance to them. And I'm just an extra pair of hands to the tribe. Nobody will miss me."

She explained their indifference to her like she was stating the color of her shirt. No emotion, no feeling, facts she'd accepted long ago.

"You could've left any time you wanted to, why now? Why with us?" Kiyahe asked.

"I wouldn't really belong anywhere else, now would I? I can't just jump into any tribe I want. And…I don't know, I just feel a pull towards you guys. To Kaya. I want to help you. I feel like maybe I could have a purpose with you."

For the first time I'd seen, Aiyana's guard faltered, and her expression was soft. She wasn't just looking for an escape, she was looking for a *purpose,* for somewhere to *belong.* It was the same reason I had wanted Kiyahe to take me to his tribe when I'd first ran into him. I felt the pull towards them inside of me and I knew that that was where I needed to go. That drive was reflected in her eyes.

"It couldn't hurt for me to have more protection," I turned to Kiyahe.

He watched her, considering.

"Can you shoot?" he asked.

She wrinkled her nose "I can shoot ok, but I throw knives even better."

Everyone's eyebrows rose in surprise, no doubt my main protector was going to make her prove the skill she claimed. I trusted she wasn't bluffing and whispered to Kiyahe again.

"It could be very useful, she can carry knives discreetly, and have them ready at all times."

Kiyahe considered some more.

"Prove it, let's go outside and see what you got," he said.

Aiyana nodded, the hint of a smile playing at the edge of her mouth. I was right, she wasn't bluffing. In fact, she seemed more than confident in her skill.

We did some target practice outside then, shooting and throwing until our hands were numb. Kiyahe with his grandfather's revolver, I with my bow and arrows, Aiyana with her knives, and the twins with extra pistols. The twins tried to hustle Aiyana and throw her off, but she threw straight and true every time, totally focused. Her skill was more than enough to be considered an asset, but she insisted that with more practice, she could do even better.

"Alright," Kiyahe said when we came back inside and shrugged out of our coats, gloves, and hats. "She's worth bringing along but it's ultimately up to Marie."

"Welcome aboard," I smiled as I held out my hand to her. She shook it and smiled back.

"But," I said, "I want you to talk it over with your family first, I don't want them pissed at me for running off with you and not telling them."

"No problem," Aiyana said.

We stayed a few hours later than planned so we could eat lunch with the Sioux and Aiyana could ask for permission to leave. Her uncle granted her request with no qualms and I gained another protector. None of the boys were thrilled about our new addition but they never complained. I was glad to have Aiyana along, the amount of testosterone on the bus greatly overpowered the estrogen and now it would feel a little more balanced. Aiyana slept in the bunk room by herself, the twins on their couches, and Kiyahe and I in the bedroom. And despite all the teasing the twins gave us, Kiyahe and I were not taking that next step just yet.

Let us form one body, one heart, and defend to the last warrior our country, our homes, our liberty, and the graves of our fathers.

–Chief Tecumseh, Shawnee.

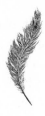

Chapter Twelve

None of us had ever been outside of the United States before.

The drive through North Dakota was long and rugged. There seemed to be a little bit of everything in regards to scenery: fields, hills, cliffs, craggy peaks, trees, scabland, grassy stretches. It had all gone brown and grey with winter setting in but there was still beauty in it. It was simple, quiet, sleepy. We passed more herds of buffalo and horses than we did towns and country houses.

"We're about a half mile from the border," Shilah announced as the bus started to buck and rumble over the crumbling road beneath us.

I sat up straighter and looked out the window, stupidly expecting to see gates with lights and border patrol officers on duty. I even had a moment of panic realizing that I didn't have a passport. But there were no lights and no border patrol people. Just the cement remains of the ports of entry and the tattered Canadian and American flags atop them, whipping wildly in the wind. It was just another ghostly, empty area. We drove through one of the ports without even stopping.

Borders would be one of many things we would have to think about once all the tribes were united and we were rebuilding our nation. Would we rebuild the old borders or create new ones in different places? Would we funnel and control the amount of people who came to our land or would we build giant walls to keep them out? It was apparent that the number one thing the tribes were worried about was losing their land again. How far would we go to protect it? How far would we go to be open and neighborly?

We stopped at a gas station just short of a mile south of the Blackfoot reservation. While the boys made camp, fueled up the bus, and replaced empty propane tanks with full ones from the gas station, Aiyana and I retreated to my bedroom to talk.

"So how much farther do you have to go until you can go home?" she asked as she looked out the window.

I picked at my fingernails while we talked, "We've visited ten tribes in a little over two months, we have seven tribes left to visit and less than a month to get it done."

"You're behind schedule then," she observed. "What happens if you're not back in a month?"

"Kiyahe's father might give us and extra week or so, but then he'll send members from the tribe out to find us," I answered. "Or find out what happened to us."

She considered, "He really thinks people might try to kill you?"

"Some have already tried," I whispered as I thought of Kalona and the determination in his hands when they'd been wrapped around my throat.

"And if you died, we would die too?" Aiyana asked quietly, finally turning to look at me.

I returned her gaze, "That's what the legend says anyway. The people get one more chance to learn to get along and act as one to protect what they love most; their families, their homes, their way of life. If they can't learn to stand together, they'll fall."

Aiyana nodded, understanding but looking worried. "It isn't easy for us. Centuries of conquering and fighting and losing. Generation after generation of grudges and bloodshed."

I listened quietly to her evaluation. As much as I *felt* like one of them, as much as I *wanted* to belong, I couldn't deny that I wasn't born and raised like they had been. I didn't have that bloody history running through my veins.

But that was why I was different. I saw the world through different eyes. I had to get them to see it too. For their sake. For mine.

"What do you think Kiyahe's parents will think of you two being together?" Aiyana changed the subject then.

I sighed, "I can only hope that they'll see it as we do. That I'm the next intended shaman for their tribe and that Kiyahe and I were meant to be together. And that we love each other. I keep thinking that when we get home, even though my job as Kaya isn't over, they'll see that when Kiyahe and I work together, we can do anything."

"What do you think *your* parents would think of it?"

I blinked, the question taking me off guard. I had never considered whether my own parents would approve. Ultimately, it didn't matter because they were dead. But if they were here, just for a moment, what would they say about me and Kiyahe?

I took a deep breath, "I think if they knew how happy he makes me, how deeply I need him, they would be happy for me. I can never be sure though, they're gone, and I don't have anything to reference it with." I smiled sheepishly, "I never even had a boyfriend to introduce them to."

Aiyana laughed, and we launched into a conversation about boys and I listened to her much more extensive dating history.

That night we all crammed into the booth on the bus and played cards and talked of trivial things. Aiyana was still sarcastic and canny, but her bitter attitude was not quite as strong as usual. I guessed it was owed to her newfound freedom and long-awaited acceptance. The twins loosened up some around her and took to teasing her, leaving Kiyahe and I to sneak glances at each other and hold hands underneath the table without being harassed.

We went to bed earlier than usual, Kiyahe saying he wanted everyone to be well rested before we hiked to the Blackfoot reservation tomorrow. But I knew the truth, Kiyahe and I's favorite part of the day now was at night when we could be alone and hold each other. The heat from the bare skin of his chest, the glint of the moonlight in his eyes, the tickle of his breath in my ear, and the melodic sound of his laugh drove me crazy with a desire I struggled to suppress. I asked him that night if it was as hard for him to control himself as it was for me and he told me it was a thousand times harder.

I doubted that.

I'd never thought of myself as beautiful, only average, simple. But Kiyahe fervently disagreed. My lank brown hair, according to him, was as soft as silk and as rich as chestnut. My dull, grey-blue eyes he compared to the stormy blue of the sky in a thunderstorm. And my translucent, pasty skin he insisted was beautifully smooth and the color of the moon. I didn't believe any of those things, but it was nice to hear them and it made me happy to see him happy.

That night I awoke from another foreshadowing dream and found myself wrapped in Kiyahe's strong arms. It wasn't a good dream and it churned my stomach knowing that the Blackfoot would not take well to us the next day, but I closed my eyes and fell back asleep in less than a few minutes in my protector's embrace.

The next day I hiked to the Blackfoot reservation with three protectors instead of my usual two. Aiyana, Neka, Kiyahe, and I met with the Blackfoot who were, as I'd feared since my dream the night before, not especially happy to see us or hear what we had to say. They were a modest sized tribe and their concern about us wasn't in believing what we were saying but in knowing which tribes had joined our alliance. Specifically, the Cheyenne, Crow, and Sioux were not their fondest neighbors and they worried about joining forces with their old enemies. Their chief and the elders decided to let us plead our case to the entire tribe and then hold a vote. We spent the rest of the day talking to, and helping out, the Blackfoot people. That night the votes were cast and counted.

We won a majority of the vote which included the chief and half of the elders. The other half of the elders and the chief's wife and daughter did not vote to join our alliance. Although there was clear dissension and tension among their leaders, Kiyahe would not let us stay longer to try and appease the nay-sayers. He insisted we had to keep moving and I relented, promising myself that we would go back and spend more time with them in the future. We left the next day for Michigan.

The tribe we were visiting in Michigan was not large nor one of the most renowned. In fact, it was only a slightly bigger grouping of our own, the Potawatomie. Michigan and the Great Lakes region was where my new tribe, my people, had originated before they were forced from their lands all those years ago. The newly formed group in the larger, southern portion of Michigan was a combination of Potawatomi descendants from all over. Most of them had drifted apart from the tribe anytime between their forced removal in the 1800s up until just before the disaster. And since the disaster, they had travelled from near and far to rejoin their people in their original lands. And, like our branch in Oklahoma, none of them had lost a loved one in the disaster. Instead of losing members, their tribe had only grown over the past few months. The absence of loss and the sense of kinship with their distant brothers and sisters led them to welcome us like old friends and agree to join our alliance wholeheartedly.

One of their young men, a charismatic and handsome boy named Jolon, played tour guide for us while we were there. Jolon was practically a Native prince charming with his good looks and magnetic charm. Unlike many other attractive men we'd met along the way, Jolon didn't flaunt his appealing qualities. He was humble and far more interested in learning about others than talking about himself.

Jolon was a tall and strong twenty-year-old who had the energy and playfulness of a child. His chestnut colored skin was a shade darker than Kiyahe's and his matte black hair hung in a single braid down to the middle of his back. His eyes were a deep onyx, the same color as the arrowhead that hung from a leather string around his neck. His face was soft, his smile wide, his eyes almost always sparkling with curiosity and interest. He was adventurous, and our arrival sparked an excitement in him that he couldn't control, and we couldn't resist.

Less than an hour after meeting him, I concluded that I was not attracted to him in any romantic way. Part of the reason was because I couldn't imagine being with anyone else now that Kiyahe and I were an obvious, and very happy, couple. I was consumed with my protector, and I didn't want anyone else but him. The other part was that Jolon reminded me of the big brother I'd never had. He was playful and carefree and his attitude towards me was the same as mine towards him. We came to like each other as friends, as siblings almost, but nothing more.

Once I had told Kiyahe what I thought and how I felt about Jolon, he put his reservations away and allowed Jolon to befriend him. Jolon showed his brotherly affection to Kiyahe and the twins, all of whom returned the comradery.

Aiyana, who at first crossed her arms and rolled her eyes at Jolon's friendliness, warmed up to his charms too. She admitted to me one afternoon while we helped the women weave baskets that she liked Jolon.

"I think he likes you too," I smiled at her. She rolled her eyes, but I couldn't help but notice the corners of her mouth threatening to form a hopeful smile. We all watched as the awkward beginning stages of romance began to unfold between Aiyana and Jolon. Kiyahe and I tentatively helped them along and offered advice while the twins teased Aiyana relentlessly. She held her own against their battery of mischievous taunting and I was grateful their new victim was better at fighting it than I was.

We spent more time with the Michigan Potawatomi than we should have, and no one wanted to leave when Kiyahe halfheartedly insisted on our departure.

The night before we were to leave, Jolon asked if he could accompany us as another protector for Kaya.

"I'll do everything you ask, and I promise I won't cause any trouble!" he begged me.

Unlike Aiyana, Jolon was a crown jewel of his tribe and I didn't want to tear him away from his people. Although he would never have a formal title of leadership, everyone loved him for his optimism and his charm, his helpfulness and his selflessness. I worried that the men wouldn't appreciate us taking away their best fisherman, and that the women would hate me for swiping their most eligible bachelor.

Jolon talked with the chief and shaman for over two hours before emerging from their lodge. The moonlight illuminated his wide, bright smile as he told us that he'd been given their blessing to accompany us. He spent a final night with his people, packing his things and bidding them goodbye. And by the morning he was on the bus with us on our way to New York.

It was a long, two-day journey to the Mohawk reservation in Northern New York. We drove along the outside of Lake Erie for much of the first day, looking out the windows at the water that stretched all the way to the horizon. Empty boats bobbed in the waves like floating headstones. The second day we inched our way through cities and towns that had been reduced to rubble like all the others. The further east we travelled, the older and grander the houses and buildings were. Structures that had stood for hundreds of years were now rickety remains of what they had once been.

And then, as we left the old cities behind and cut through the northern part of the state, it was as if we'd been transported back in time to the western part of the country. Dense forests filled with hundreds, maybe even thousands of trees surrounded us. Winter had already settled in here, the immense forests covered in pristine white blankets of glistening snow. Although it was warm and cozy in the bus, I shivered at the sight of the cold snow. There were tribes and individuals who had been used to heated houses and fireplaces that were now bunking down or travelling through the wintry season. Part of me worried about how they would survive in the blistering cold while the other part of me believed that if their ancestors had done it, then they could too.

Whether it was the biting cold or their history of having been fur traders, the Mohawk people kept nice and warm with their abundant number of pelts. They used the furs for coats over their clothing, insulation in their longhouses, and blankets for bedding. A large fire burned outside of their main longhouse while inside fireplaces, wood burning stoves, and longhouse fire pits kept their residents warm. The whole reservation seemed to glow with warmth and light.

Unfortunately, their perception of us wasn't as warm as their homes were. The Mohawk were well separated, well distanced from their Native neighbors and weren't concerned with joining any alliances. They also fervently swore that they would be far more careful than their ancestors had been with who they trusted and allowed on their land the next time outsiders came up on their shores. It took hours of discussion to finally convince them to join our alliance. They weren't thrilled, and their letter of promise was bare bones and unenthusiastic. But we could count on them as allies all the same.

Before we left New York, I started coming on with a cold. Like he did with almost everything, Kiyahe overreacted and thought I should see a doctor or a healer and that we should stay with the Mohawk until I got better. But I insisted that I was fine and would be over it soon. We needed to keep moving if we were going to make it back before Ahote's deadline. During the long drive southwest, to Kentucky, I tried to stifle my coughs and hold back my shivers as much as possible. I gave in and took medicine before Kiyahe could practically shove it down my throat. After a while longer, I excused myself to the bedroom to take a nap, thinking I just needed more rest. I hacked a few violent coughs into my pillow to stifle the noise and covered up with every blanket we had in the bedroom before succumbing to the drowsy effects of the medicine.

I woke up in the middle of the night with Kiyahe softly snoring next to me. While I stared up at the ceiling, I realized that I must have slept through the rest of the drive to Kentucky. I was a little miffed that no one had bothered to wake me to eat and plan our trip to the Shawnee reservation. I had a cold for crying out loud, not pneumonia. I quietly got up and ghosted out of the room, through the bunk room where Aiyana and Jolon were sleeping, and into the living area where the twins snored loudly on their couches.

Fighting against the tickle of a cough in my throat, I went through the cupboards until I found more medicine, making sure to take non-drowsy pills this time. As the pallid moonlight barely penetrated through the blinds on the bus, I made my way back to bed, waiting for dawn and stifling my coughs and sneezes into my pillow so that I wouldn't wake Kiyahe.

The next day we hiked the half mile to the Shawnee reservation and I could tell the cold medicine wasn't helping. I was sluggish and slow, my legs feeling tired and my lungs rasping with mucous. I had to ask the twins, Jolon, and Kiyahe to slow down for me more than once. I was jealous of Aiyana, who was staying with the bus that day. I never got the option of staying back and taking a day off.

A woman with a baby strapped to her back took us to her neighbor's, where the Shawnee chief was helping several other men re-roof the house. I must have looked as bad as I felt because Kiyahe did most of the talking for me and the chief looked at me like I was a zombie. When Kiyahe finished, the Shawnee chief said he would gather the elders and discuss the matter. Before he left to do so, though, he suggested that we let him escort us to their healer so that I could have hot tea with herb roots. Kiyahe accepted the offer before I could protest that I was fine. I didn't have the energy or the patience to really fight it, and hot tea sounded better and better as we walked through the chill to the healer's house.

The tea did help, it warmed my insides and helped me stifle my cough. I drank three more cups before the chief returned to tell us that the tribe had decided to join our alliance. Maybe it was the herbs in the tea or maybe it was another successful alliance formed, but I was feeling a little better when we left the Shawnee reservation.

The next day we made the short drive to Tennessee and while the ugly greenish grey clouds swirled overhead, hinting at a winter storm, I took the absolute max amount of cold medicine that I could take without overdosing.

The night before we were to meet the Cherokee tribe, I had another prophetic dream. It started out with a memory, just like all the others. It was a cold, snowy day and me and my cousins were trying to dig a tunnel through a big snowdrift in my cousin's backyard. After all the breaks we'd taken to have snowball fights and eat the snow, we'd finally made a tunnel big enough for our eight-year-old selves to squeeze through. We took turns worming our way through the tunnel, laughing the entire time. It was my second time through the tunnel when the pile came crashing down on me, burying me in the icy darkness. I screamed and cried while my cousins tried to dig me out. Someone went and got my dad and he managed to grab me by my boots and yank me out of the snow. He told me not to cry as he wiped snow out of my eyelashes and tears off my face. After I'd calmed down, we played King of the Mountain on top of the snow instead of digging tunnels underneath it.

The dream repeated up until the part when the snow pile buried me. Only the second time, no one was there to unbury me or pull me out. I screamed as the snow continued to press on me and I couldn't breathe. My chest was being crushed, there was no air left in the tunnel, and I began to see red and feel nothing but ice all around me.

A raspy gasp escaped my throat as I was jolted awake. The sound of a raging blizzard screamed outside the bus, the wind rocking us side to side, the old bus creaking in protest. I laid there in bed while a fit of racking coughs seized me and while I tried to regain my breath, I could see white plumes of air coming from my mouth and nose in the dark. I couldn't feel my toes or my fingers and it took me a while to realize that the shaking of the bed was from my violent shivering. I tried to say Kiyahe's name, but it came out quieter than a whisper. I listened to the bus continue its creaky complaints.

It took several more minutes and a loud gust of wind to get Kiyahe to wake up. I was too frozen to roll over and look at him, but I could hear him cuss under his breath at the frigid temperature of our bedroom. He said my name, but I was too cold and tired to move or answer. Then he started shouting my name and shaking me. When his beautiful blue eyes came into my line of sight I managed to blink at him but nothing else. My body felt like it was still trapped in the snow pile and it was all I could do to keep breathing.

Kiyahe flew around the bus then, slamming doors open, flipping on lights, and yelling at everyone to get up. He shouted at Aiyana and Jolon to get me warm while he and the twins went out into the storm to figure out why the propane heat had stopped working.

As I laid there stiff and frozen, Aiyana told Jolon to gather up all the blankets from the beds and cupboards while she shut the bedroom door and stripped down to her underwear. I wanted to ask her what the hell she was doing but my lips were too frozen to speak. She only allowed time for one shiver to coarse through her before throwing the covers off of me and removing my clothes as well. My confusion and fear must have shown because she explained to me as she stripped me down to my underwear.

"We have to get your body heat up and I can do that faster if I don't have to heat our clothes up too."

As I drifted in and out of consciousness, Aiyana jumped into bed with me, throwing the covers over the top of us. She pushed me onto my side, and hugged me from behind, throwing a leg over mine and wrapping her arms around my torso, pinning my arms inside her grasp. My body must have been significantly colder than hers because she cussed under her breath at my chill and she felt like she was on fire to me. I realized it must be my illness that was rendering me so useless compared to the rest of them.

Jolon came in the bedroom then and began layering us with blankets. When he ran out of those he piled pillows on and around us, trying to pack our heat in like a blanket igloo. When he was finished burying us under the mountain of bedding, he suited up and joined the other guys outside.

Aiyana was telling me it would be ok as she rubbed her hands up and down my arms, trying to heat me up with friction. A rough cough full of mucous gripped me then and I hacked into my pillow shaking Aiyana with me. I coughed until the mucous left my lungs and oozed out onto my pillow. It was warm and wet.

And red.

Through my peripherals I watched the red blood stain my pillow and felt my head swim.

That was when I blacked out.

Perhaps they are not stars, but rather openings in heaven where the love of our lost ones pours through and shines down upon us to let us know they are happy.

—Native American quote.

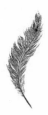

Chapter Thirteen

I woke to find my pillow changed and Aiyana replaced by Kiyahe in the blanket cocoon with me. Kiyahe told me a wire connection in the bus had gone bad and that that was why we had no heat. It wasn't something he could quickly fix, he would need tools that he didn't have. He also said we would have to wait out the storm in the bus until morning, when he could carry me to the Cherokee reservation and have a healer tend to me. Aiyana, Jolon, and the twins stayed in my room with us with the door shut. Every bit of body heat was packed into one room not just to thaw me out but to keep everyone else warm too. I was watching Jolon rub his hands together to keep them warm when I blacked out again.

The next time I woke it was still dark. Seeing me conscious, Aiyana tried to spoon feed me some cough syrup. Just as I was trying to swallow the second spoonful, a fit of coughing overcame me, and I spit the liquid back out onto her face. Neka busted up with laughter and Shilah hid his smile behind his hand while I tried to apologize to Aiyana. My mouth moved slowly, and the words were silent as she waved off my apology and wiped her face with the back of her sweatshirt sleeve. I blacked out again shortly after that.

When dawn finally came, I flickered in and out of consciousness with furious speed.

Kiyahe started barking orders, blackness.

The blankets were removed from me, blackness.

I questioned why I couldn't feel the cold while someone dressed me, blackness.

I was bundled and being cradled in someone's arms, blackness.

The wind shrieked while someone ran with me, blackness.

The line between conscious and unconscious was so blurry that I couldn't tell what was real and what wasn't. The next time I woke, I was in a lodge with a roaring fire blazing in the middle of the dirt floor. Incense burned all around me and the hazy smoke made me drowsy. I was wrapped in what felt like buckskin or furs, I couldn't look down to be sure. My eyes, burdened by heavy eyelids, were focused on the fire and my violent shivering rocked the cot underneath me. I was alone in the room but Kiyahe was not far, I could hear him arguing with someone in another language outside the door. For once I was too weak to worry about what would happen next.

I dreamt that I was walking along a rushing river in late spring. On the side where I was walking, the field was flat and grassy, punctuated occasionally by large, hardwood trees that were flushed in green. Flowers of all different shapes and colors were in full bloom and insects flew between them, creating a constant buzz that was a background noise to the many birds singing in the tree tops. It was a beautiful melody and I smiled at the sweet sound of it while the sunlight warmed my face, arms, legs, and bare feet.

I was vaguely aware that this was not another of my prophetic dreams. It was different; I had no memory of this place, no confusion, no need to understand.

Everything was perfect, and I was calm. A calm I had never experienced before.

The river ran full and fast, the current tumbling over the rocks underneath. The light reflected off of rainbow trout in an array of colors as they swished their way downstream. I stopped to dip my toes in the crystal-clear stream, it was chilly. The water had probably melted from the snowy mountaintops that were barely visible in the distance behind me. When summer came, the water would be warmer. On the other side of the river were sheer cliff sides the color of rust. Sporadic holes punctuated the the length of the cliff face, homes for snakes, mice, and other creatures. For a moment I was jealous of them, they had such a beautiful view outside their front doors. Atop one of the cliffs stood an elk, looking down on the beautiful valley with a robust chest and wise eyes.

After about a hundred yards, I caught sight of a companion from my first journey. I was overjoyed to see the wolf. My memories of him had not done him justice. His fur was so white and pure that it nearly glowed in the bright sunshine. His aquamarine eyes glistened a pale blue like the rushing water beside me. He ran straight for me and I dropped to my knees laughing and crying. He plowed into me, nearly knocking me over, barking his throaty bark, nuzzling me with his large snout, and licking my face with his long tongue. After our reunion, he walked beside me, his large head parallel with the height of my ribcage and his large paws more than twice the width of my own bare feet.

I knew I was dreaming when the man started speaking to me. At first, I thought the deep, grandfatherly voice was coming from the wolf, but when I looked at my companion's face, his mouth was doing nothing more than panting and smiling that toothy grin. As the voice spoke, I looked around me to find out where it was coming from and saw no one.

"You are doing well, Kaya. I always knew you would."

"Who said that?" I shouted the question, my command shaky and fearful. My head whipped around to find the source of the man's voice.

The man chuckled, "Be calm, my daughter. You will not, and cannot, be harmed here."

My eyes kept searching as I walked with the wolf. "Who are you?" I asked, a little more calmly this time.

"You know who I am, Marie. And I've been with you the whole time. I always will be."

Before I could form my next question, the voice continued.

"Your body is weak, but it will heal. I thought you might need something to heal your mind and your heart as well.

As I came around a bend in the stream, the sight ahead set my heart throbbing and my eyes watering. My parents stood in the sunshine, holding hands, waiting for me.

I ran to them, my feet flying and my heart pounding. Like the wolf, I ran full speed into their arms, letting their solidness stop me. My mother and father surrounded and embraced me, the three of us crying and laughing. All the words I didn't get a chance to say before the disaster came pouring out of my mouth in a flood of emotion.

"I'm so sorry I didn't get to tell you goodbye! I love you and I appreciate you and I can't believe you're here! I've missed you so much!"

"We love you too, Marie. You've done so well, and we couldn't be more proud of you!" my mother smiled through her tears.

"I've felt so alone sometimes," I sobbed.

"You've never been alone, Marie. We've always been watching, and God's always been there. And you have great friends and a devoted protector," my dad reminded me.

I nodded, knowing he was right. Even in the beginning, during that first journey when I'd felt the most alone, I had had the wolf, who now yipped and panted beside us, wanting to be a part of the attention too.

The three of us, still wrapped in each other's arms, laughed through our tears and knelt to pet the wolf.

The man spoke again in his wise and clear voice. "You have to go back now Kaya. There are still more trials for you to go through and I need you to be strong. I need you to *believe*, my daughter. Can you do that?"

I choked back a sob, realizing that I could not stay, and my parents could not come with me. I nodded my head, trying to be brave. "I will do everything in my power to help the people. I will believe that you are all with me."

I committed the warmth of the sunshine and my parents embrace to memory before I awoke.

My time in the dream had seemed so brief, but in reality, I had been unconscious for two days while my body battled the fever. I awoke to find Kiyahe sitting by my bedside, his head bowed in prayer. Tentatively, I reached out and put my hand on the warm skin of his shoulder. He sighed before looking up at me.

"Thank God. I thought I was going to lose you," he whispered brokenly. For once, his eyes weren't the bright and brilliant blue I had come to know and love. They were a dark and murky blue, lackluster and a bit crazed looking. His eyes looked like they had sunk back in his head and they were surrounded by deep purplish circles. The rich bronze glow of his skin seemed paled and sickly. I had never seen my strong protector look so haggard and vulnerable.

I managed a weak smile for him, "I'm not going anywhere. We have a job to do."

He chuckled softly, "Always so stubborn."

"I think it's a side effect from being around you," I teased.

"Well I wouldn't have you any other way," he smiled then, brightly and fully. My heart stuttered at the sight of it.

A woman entered the lodge then, letting a gust of cold air in with her. I shivered once and Kiyahe tucked the furry blanket tighter around me. The woman quickly and gracefully approached us, shooing Kiyahe away from my cot. He moved aside without argument.

The woman looked to be in her late thirties or early forties, her loose black hair slightly graying at the roots and sprinkled with snowflakes from outside. Her small dark eyes were quick and they flitted across me, taking notes of my condition. Besides her eyes, everything else about her was small too. Her height, her size, her nose, mouth, and chin. Even her hands, one of which she put to my forehead to take my temperature, were small. I felt like I was in a cozy mouse hole and she was a mother mouse, taking care of me.

She flitted to the middle of the room where a pot hung over the fire. "My name is Sihu," she said as she removed the pot from above the flames. "I'm the shaman and the chief of this Cherokee tribe."

I blinked, confused, "You're the shaman *and the chief?*" My voice crackled slightly, and I had to clear my throat, I was still sick, though not as severely as when I'd first arrived.

"Yes," Sihu answered. "My husband died in the disaster and I do not have any children."

I felt a wave of sympathy for this woman. She had lost her husband and now had no family at all. She was alone, and the full responsibility of the tribe was on her shoulders. Why she was taking the time to tend to me I did not know. Didn't they have a healer for that?

Sihu answered my question before I could ask it. "We lost our healer and all of our elders as well. The drought and the heat of the fires burned up our crops and most of our homes. We lost many people."

Sihu poured the hot water over some leaves in a chipped coffee mug and stirred the mixture. "This will help your body drive the poison out faster," she said.

"Poison?" I asked.

"Yes. When Kiyahe brought you in he thought you had a flu of some sort but then I noticed your veins. They were protruding and swollen, and they were purple and black in color. I suspected someone had poisoned you and I've been purging your body for the last two days to try and rid you of it. So far, it's been working well, though I have to admit it's been years since I went to medical school so I'm a bit rusty."

Sihu helped me sit up and I wasn't sure if it was the movement or this newfound knowledge that someone had tried to kill me again that made me dizzy.

"Now drink this, I will go tell your friends you are awake now," Sihu said as she handed me the brew before she flitted out the door and into the cold. The drink smelled terrible, so I downed it in as few gulps as I could.

"I think it was the Mohawk," Kiyahe said when we were alone and I'd finished the brew. "Sihu said the poison was enough to kill you but not enough to do it quickly. I think they slipped it in something you ate or drank just before we left so that you wouldn't die when we were with them. So that it would look like you died of a flu while we were with a different tribe." Kiyahe ground his teeth together and the crazed, burning look returned to his eyes.

"You can't know that for sure," I rationalized. "They weren't our biggest fans, but they still joined our alliance."

"Joining us could have been a ruse. Something to satisfy you and to get us to leave. Killing you could have given them an out from allying with us."

It was clear Kiyahe had thought out his theory thoroughly, but it was still just a theory. Though I had to admit the Mohawk were the most recent tribe we had visited that did not particularly like us, we couldn't be sure that it was them who had tried to kill me. And throwing around accusations wasn't going to keep our alliances intact.

"The next time I visit them I won't eat or drink anything that's offered to me. And I'll bring even more protectors if I need to," I said.

"Next time? No, Marie. I'm not going to let you go there again, it's too dangerous," Kiyahe swore.

"I'll have to touch base with our allies for the rest of my life, Kiyahe. That's what a good leader does. You can't prove they were the ones who tried to kill me, and you can't keep me from going," I told him, my voice rising with anger.

"You promised me you would try to be more careful," he said in a low voice, trying to keep his own temper in check.

"I am. I will. And you promised you would try to trust me more."

Kiyahe took a big breath and we sat there in silence, thinking about our promises and how they weren't the easiest ones to keep.

Our silent reveries were interrupted by another blast of cold air as Aiyana, Jolon, and Neka entered the lodge to see me. The three of them smiled from ear to ear at the sight of me, conscious and sitting up in bed. I couldn't help but smile back at them.

"Thank God you're alive!" Neka shouted. "I thought you were going to leave me with the disgusting lovebirds and Negative Nancy over there, and my pain in the ass brother. So unfair, Kaya. And when we're so close to going home!"

I laughed, "I couldn't leave my favorite twin! What would Shilah do without me?!" Everyone bursted with laughter except Neka who rolled his eyes and ever so gently punched me mockingly on the arm. "Glad to have you back, girl," he said.

"Seriously, there's been a major testosterone overload without you around," Aiyana said in her usual sarcastic voice. She came over to my cot, Jolon in tow behind her.

Everyone put in their two cents as they filled me in on what I had missed the last two days. Kiyahe had been the one to run with me in his arms through the snowstorm to the edge of the reservation, nearly catching frostbite in the process. His unwavering loyalty and need to protect me made my heart swell with love and I forgot about our little tiff earlier. Kiyahe had pounded on the door of the first lodge he'd found and I had been taken to Sihu immediately. While I'd been healing, my protectors had been bunking next door with good friends of Sihu's and playing the part of good helpers with the tribe. While they'd been working their tails off and promoting Kaya, Kiyahe had almost never left my side.

"Sihu put the fate of our alliance to a vote and everyone voted to join," Kiyahe said proudly. "It seems that nomads have been spreading the word of Kaya and you have quite a good reputation. The Cherokee had heard of you before we'd even arrived."

I smiled, remembering the nomad we'd met in Nebraska. Dyani had promised to spread word and I wondered just how far my message had spread since then.

"As much as they like you though," Aiyana piped in, "We worked our asses off winning you votes while you sat here threatening to ditch us. So, you're welcome."

Kiyahe rolled his eyes at her, "*Anyway*, we can get moving as soon as your better. We just have Georgia and Mississippi left to go."

"And then we're home!" Neka threw his hands up in excitement.

I felt my face light up in a smile at the thought of going back home. I would get to see Mahala and Hiawassee and the rest of my new tribe very soon. But then my eyes caught Kiyahe's and I saw my concerns mirrored in them. Would his parents and the tribe accept me as the next shaman and Kiyahe's future companion? Would the tribes we'd visited stay true to our alliance while we were gone? Would we be able to rebuild a nation of united people?

"It will be good to be home," Kiyahe said, his smile small. He was trying to be optimistic, trying to ease my worries.

Sihu returned then and shooed everyone out, saying I needed to rest and heal. Kiyahe kissed me on my still slightly fevered forehead before begrudgingly leaving with the others. Sihu made me eat a hunk of cornbread and drink another cup of the foul-tasting brew before re-tucking the blankets around me and instructing me to sleep.

But I had slept for two days straight and I wasn't tired in the slightest. I watched her from the cot as she pulled a rocking chair close to the fire and stoked the logs to get them blazing again. Then she grabbed a basket from under her bed and sat with it by the fire. The basket was filled with what looked like bark shavings and dried grasses. As I watched, her small and nimble fingers began to weave the shavings and grasses into a bowl shape.

"What are you making?" I asked her from my cot.

"A basket dear girl, go to sleep now," she instructed from her chair, her eyes trained studiously on the creation between her hands.

"What will you use it for?" I prodded. Despite the sweet-smelling incense wafting through the lodge and the coziness of the warm fire, I didn't feel even the slightest urge to go back to sleep.

Sihu sighed, seeing that I would not rest for some time. "I don't know yet," she answered.

"Do you all weave baskets? Your tribe?" I asked.

"No. Do you all ask so many questions? Your tribe?" she asked pointedly, a smile spreading across her soft face, crinkling the crow's feet at the corners of her eyes.

I smiled back, "I wouldn't know, I'm usually the one asking the questions. Kiyahe gets annoyed with it but I can't help it. This is a totally different world for me."

Sihu finally turned in her chair to look at me, her hands still busying themselves with the basket. She must have had many years of practice to be able to weave so effortlessly without looking. "It's a different world for all of us since the Fire Rains. But I suppose not having your family and your culture would make it even harder."

My mind flickered to my parents and the dream I'd had. I smiled again, "No, I still have my family. I just have another family now too."

The Cherokee chief looked at me, her expression bemused. Meanwhile her hands continued working the pile of shavings and grasses in her lap. I felt her question hanging in the air between us and explained, "I saw them. While I was sick. I'm not sure if it was God or the Great Spirit or whoever, but He was taking care of them. In heaven. Or someplace beautiful like that. I don't exactly know, I just know that they're safe and happy. And they said they're with me all the time. The Voice said He is with me too. Does that make any sense?"

Sihu's hands stopped moving and she stared into my soul with her eyes. At first, I worried that I sounded crazy, maybe I was since I'd been poisoned after all. I started to wonder if maybe the dream had been nothing more than just that. A dream. But then I stopped myself. No, it was real. I had seen and talked to my parents and I had felt the truth of the experience in my core. I couldn't explain why or how but I knew in my heart that my parents and God or the Great Spirit were with me.

"You're not sure if it was God or the Great Spirit?" she finally asked.

Her question was not what I had been expecting. "Uhm… no, I don't. I mean, I heard Him. I know He was there. But I guess I don't know exactly what to call Him." I grimaced at my response, I sounded like such an idiot.

"Why does it matter what you call Him?" she asked.

"I'm sorry?"

"You know He was there and you believe what He said. What else matters? You think He would drop you like a stone in a river if you called Him by the wrong title?"

"No, I just… I don't want to be disrespectful and call Him by the wrong name."

She snorted, "I think He has more important concerns than what name you call Him by. Listen girl, every culture has different names and different titles for Him. Do you think they're all going to hell or someplace terrible because they got His name wrong?"

I shook my head, "No, I wouldn't think so. There are countless good people around the world, it shouldn't matter as long as they believe."

Sihu nodded her approval, "I think you are right, Kaya. *Believing* is the point. Believing is the most important. As long as you believe He is with you, you are always loved. You are always home."

I smiled, "That sounds about right to me."

One of the things my parents taught me, and I'll always be grateful for the gift, is to not ever let anybody else define me.

—Wilma Mankiller, Cherokee.

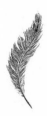

Chapter Fourteen

It felt strange to be leaving the Cherokee tribe so soon, considering I had been unconscious for most of my visit. But as soon as I was able to walk and feed myself, Sihu and Kiyahe saw no reason why I couldn't travel. We bid the Cherokee goodbye and promised to return someday so that I could spend more time with the people who had voted to support me, without knowing much more than my name.

Two days later we arrived in Georgia to meet the Creek tribe. And we soon learned that the Creek were nothing short of interesting. For starters, they had two chiefs, a phenomenon I had not yet seen and Kiyahe had never heard of. The seventeen-year-old twin brothers had lost their parents in the disaster and their father had not had the chance to hold the ceremony that would announce which of his sons would serve as the next chief. So, they had agreed to co-lead the tribe and to let any of their disputed decisions be decided by the tribal elders.

Their wives, one my age and the other a couple years older had also split the duties typically given to a chief's wife. The older wife had been gifted with visions, and so she served as the shaman while the other was a phenomenal healer who not only had a special touch but had completed medical school and previously worked as a nurse. Although they were young and new to their positions, the four of them were close knit and worked together like a well-oiled machine. They were also highly respected by their tribe. We got along with them wonderfully and in less than a few hours, had added them to our list of allies.

Jolon had opted to stay at the bus so that Neka and Shilah could spend time with the twin chiefs who had befriended them from the start. While the two sets of twins bonded through hunting and fishing, Aiyana and I spent time with the wives while Kiyahe watched from over by the door of the lodge. Aiyana and the older wife sewed blankets by the fire while the younger wife taught me about brews, incense, herbs, and medicine. She was a great teacher, combining science and ancient tradition in her explanations of what to use and why for different ailments. I focused intently on everything she told me, committing her lessons to memory. When we got back to the Potawatomi and when, *if*, I was accepted as the next shaman, I would also take on the responsibility of a healer, since both responsibilities fell on the chief's wife as per tradition of my new tribe. Part of me felt burdened with my growing list of responsibilities: uniting the tribes, leading the tribes, becoming a chief's wife, becoming a shaman, and becoming a healer. Sometimes it was all I could do not to explode.

But when I thought of God and my parents being by my side, and when I thought about being with Kiyahe, the list seemed more like a blessing than a burden. I snuck a glance at my protector while the younger chief's wife prattled about the uses for sweet grass, and smiled. Kiyahe smiled back, the firelight glinting in his eyes and my heart stuttering in arrhythmia.

The two sets of twins met up with us just before dinner and the nine of us bundled up against the softly falling snow and walked to the community building at the center of the reservation. When we walked inside I shivered against a blast of heat and squinted against the bright industrial lights that lit up the main room. Once my pupils had adjusted, I marveled at the return of modern light. The chief twin who was married to the older wife chuckled at my expression.

"I take it nobody else has electricity up and running yet, huh?"

I shook my head dumbly as I stared at the ceiling. The purple spots in my vision were telling me not to stare directly at the lights but I couldn't help myself. The world had felt so medieval, so ancient, since the disaster and the loss of lights and technology. Sure, I had seen tribes string wires from car batteries to power some small things, but nothing like this.

For the most part, it made me happy that we were overcoming the odds and returning to some level of modernity. But a small part of me felt sad and I couldn't exactly explain why.

Maybe it was because there was a strange charm to bare necessities. To discovering yourself through survival.

Or maybe it was because I had seen so many people bond together in our primitive state.

Either way I concluded that it was a good thing that we were rebuilding and moving forward, as people all over the world would soon be doing if they hadn't begun already.

The Creek held a massive feast in our honor and we ate until we couldn't eat any more and we began to feel sleepy in the large dining room of the community center. But then the sound of music pulled us out of our stupor and we joined the tribe in dancing, laughing, and talking into the night. As I'd done with every tribe, I spent the first couple hours trying to talk to as many people and shake as many hands as I could, promising to be a good leader and to take care of our newly forming nation of people. But as the older generations and young families headed home to bed, I let myself be pulled in by the energetic party goers. Kiyahe kept close to my side as we danced with the twins and Aiyana. I felt a small stab of pity for Jolon who couldn't attend the party with us and promised myself he would accompany us to our last tribe before we headed home.

It was during a slow song when the twins were twirling beautiful Creek girls around and I was wrapped in Kiyahe's strong arms that Aiyana asked for my permission to go back to Jolon at the bus. I gave her my blessing to go and when Kiyahe started to interject I silenced him with a kiss. Aiyana threw me a quick wink before slipping through the crowd and out the door into the winter night.

"I'm gonna miss this," I told Kiyahe softly as I laid my head on his shoulder. Vance Joy's, "Straight Into Your Arms," played softly from the large speakers in the room and the cozy warmth made my eyes close sleepily.

"Miss what exactly?" Kiyahe whispered into my hair.

I pulled away slightly so I could look into his turquoise eyes. The more I thought of him as mine and me as his, the easier it was to lose myself in those eyes. To feel like they would never leave me. "This trip," I answered. "The adventure, the sights, the meeting new people, the possibilities…" I shook my head, "After the disaster I prayed every day that it was all a dream. That things would go back to normal. And when I found you and the tribe and realized that that would never happen... I prayed that I would be able to settle into a new type of normal. But now I realize I don't want normalcy. I want adventure, I want possibilities. I don't want things to get boring. Because I feel so alive right now. Does that make any sense?"

Kiyahe laughed softly, the soft rumble of it reverberating in his chest and spiking my heartbeat. "Well first of all, I don't think life could ever be so blandly described as *normal* with you," he smiled. "And if I had to bet on it, I'd guess that the Great Spirit has a whole life of adventure planned for you."

"I think you're right," I said. "He told me that I would have more trials and that I needed to be strong, I just hope I don't lose myself or anyone else along the way."

"*He* told you that? Who's He?" Kiyahe asked, a small crinkle of concern forming between his raven black eyebrows. I reached up with a finger and gently smoothed it out, I didn't like his handsome face masked with worry. "God. The Great Spirit. Whatever title you want to use. I heard Him when I was..." I couldn't bring myself to use the word *dying*. The memory of the dream was so beautiful I didn't want to taint it with something as terrible as dying. Even though that was exactly what I had been doing. "when I was asleep," I finished.

Kiyahe opened his mouth to say something but then closed it again. I stretched up on my toes to kiss him, I never seemed to be able to fill my need for his touch. The electric, magnetic pull between us was unrelenting.

"Don't worry, we can make it through anything. We're not alone," I said with a soft smile, feeling the truth of my words in my heart. The faint smell of a sunshine filled meadow and the whisper of a wolf's howl reached me through the boisterous crowd. "At least... I *feel* like we can make it through anything. Especially when I have you with me."

Kiyahe stared deeply into my eyes and for a split second I worried what would happen if I was wrong, if I *didn't* have him with me. "You...you will stay with me, right?" I said so quietly I almost couldn't hear my own words.

And then that brilliant, heartwarming smile spread across his face and I knew the answer before it left his inviting lips. "I will *always* stay with you. As long as you'll have me, I'll be right here."

I nodded and answered as if he had asked it as a question. "I'll always want you with me."

He pulled me to him then, as if he couldn't stand the small distance any more than I could. Our mouths met with eagerness and we struggled to keep our embrace appropriate for public eyes.

Our declarations filled my heart with light and peace, and they temporarily alleviated the worry that had become my constant companion.

I had never been the type of girl to make careless promises left and right, I had been raised that a promise was meaningful and something you tried your hardest to keep. Since I'd met Kiyahe and his tribe, and all the other tribes since then, I had made dozens of promises.

I just hoped and prayed I could keep them all.

And I knew that I would give everything to do so.

"Do you think it's safe to go back to the bus yet?" I said breathily when we'd finally broken the kiss. I saw my desire mirrored in his eyes and for a thrilling moment I wondered if Kiyahe would take my words as an invitation. As a surrender.

But then he smiled and like the good protector and gentleman he was, he shook his head. "I think if Jolon and Aiyana have *half* the love and desire we have for each other it is nowhere *near* safe to go back to the bus," he chuckled.

I laughed with him and we danced late into the night, leaving only when a handful of partiers were left. When we returned to the bus we found Aiyana and Jolon cocooned in a blanket sleeping on one of the couches together.

"Oh, *HELL* no!" Neka nearly shouted when he saw them. Shilah and Kiyahe and I smothered his words with hushes to be quiet.

"Just sleep in the bunk room tonight, you'll be fine," I hissed at him as we tiptoed past the love birds.

"This is crap!" he hissed back. "I can *never* sleep on that couch again! They defiled it!"

"Shut up and let it go, Neka. Go to bed," Kiyahe told him sternly. Aiyana stirred in her sleep and a drowsy smile spread across her unconscious face. Neka snorted in disgust and Shilah and I couldn't help but laugh at Neka's expense. Typical Aiyana, irritating people even in her sleep.

It was a beautiful drive from Georgia to Mississippi. The rolling hills were blanketed with snow and the rushing rivers churned icy and clear throughout the countryside. The occasional decimated towns and cities that became visible around the bends in the road were blanketed with a fluffy white layer of peacefulness. They looked so quiet and serene that I was almost able to convince myself that they weren't ghost towns. That their residents were bundled up inside where it was warm and not exposed to the freezing elements in the spots where they'd perished. The delusion worked for much of the drive. And when it faltered I needed only to bury my face in my protector's shoulder and close my eyes for a few moments to avoid the sight of the graveyards. Within those few moments, the graveyards were swallowed up by the rolling hills.

Aiyana elected to stay behind while Jolon, the twins, Kiyahe, and I trudged through over a foot of snow on our way to the Choctaw reservation. By the time we arrived at their outskirts, I was more concerned with getting inside and getting warm than I was with meeting the people.

Our first mistake with the Choctaw was assuming they would be friendly.

When we had made camp the day before, less than a mile from their reservation, Kiyahe had given us the routine rundown of the tribe's history. The Choctaw had been one of the earliest to engage and work with European settlers all those years ago. Their southern lands, full of rich soil and abundant game had been greatly desired by whites because of their value. The Choctaw had dealt more in treaties than they had in battles with the Europeans but, inevitably, they were removed by force in the end. We assumed that they would be deal makers and that, with the right words and encouragement, they would be persuaded to join our alliance without too much trouble. So far, Kiyahe's knowledge of tribal histories and his father's advice had been mostly on point.

This was not one of those times.

We were escorted to a large lodge where we met their chief, Tatenga. He was a tall, strong, barrel chested man whose stern face and sharp eyes made him especially intimidating. His age was impossible to pin down but looking at the deep pockmarks in his mahogany cheeks and the angry wrinkles around his eyes, I guessed him to be in his forties or fifties. Tatenga's wife had died long ago in childbirth, Tatenga's baby boy dying with her. Despite his harsh demeanor and fierce eyes, I felt a small welling of pity for the man who had apparently spent most of his adult life alone, with no family of his own.

Tatenga wouldn't allow me to speak and did all of his talking in his Native language, leaving Kiyahe the only one able, and allowed, to speak on our behalf. I tried to look at the chief attentively but softly, not wanting to challenge him in any way. Tatenga, however, glared into my sole unwaveringly, his expression full of anger and disgust. I tried not to flinch at his obvious hatred of me.

When Kiyahe finished, the chief finally turned his gaze from me to Kiyahe and spoke a few sentences that I, of course, couldn't understand, and I knew that he did this on purpose. When the chief was finished, Kiyahe translated for us that Tatenga wanted no part of our alliance or anything to do with a white woman. I flinched, Kiyahe never did sugarcoat things for me, but I quickly regained my composure. I was used to being discriminated against and I would not let this last chief on our journey intimidate me.

"Tell him about all the other tribes we've allied with and offer him the letters to read," I told Kiyahe while keeping my gaze in the vicinity of the chief.

Our second mistake was arrogantly assuming that our vast number of allies would convince even our last acquaintance.

Kiyahe conveyed my message and the chief gave his thundering response, his booming voice filled with enough bass that it shook me to my core and I could feel my confidence slide off my face.

"Take Marie outside," Kiyahe instructed the boys. Jolon grabbed me by the elbow and pulled me toward the door while the twins backed out with us, their eyes never leaving Kiyahe and the chief.

"No, I'm not leaving without you!" I shouted as I pulled against Jolon and towards Kiyahe.

The chief boomed more words I didn't understand and waved his hand like he was swatting at a fly.

Kiyahe turned to me and I searched his face for any sign of fear or concern and found none. The worry was mine alone. "I'll be fine, he respects me as a chief's son and won't hurt me. I have to do the talking here; he's too hurt to listen to you."

Before I could ask what that meant, Jolon gave a final tug and pulled me out into the blinding snow. The twins close on our heels, the door slamming behind us.

"What does he mean the chief's hurt? He looks completely fine!" I shouted at Jolon who kept his grip on my elbow for fear I'd run back into the lodge.

"I don't know but you need to calm the hell down, Kiyahe wouldn't let you out of his sight unless it was important so just chill for a few minutes," Jolon said.

"Well she'll certainly be chilled in a few minutes," Shilah said as he rubbed his hands together in the wintry air.

"Frozen is more like it," Neka added, his breath coming out in white plumes with his words.

We huddled there like penguins in the cold, hoping someone would offer us shelter in one of their lodges but no one approached us. Everyone went about their business throwing worried sideways glances at us or throwing daggers with their eyes. The chill sinking in wasn't just from the frigid air.

After a few minutes a woman who looked to be in her early thirties approached us. But instead of offering us shelter, she started screaming at us in her Native language, which none of us understood. And unfortunately, our interpreter and my main protector was still engaged with the chief inside his lodge. At first, we pretended to ignore her, hoping she would say her piece and leave but then she raised a hand to hit me, either out of anger or to get my attention, I wasn't sure.

That was when we made our third mistake.

Neka caught her by the wrist and yelled back at her, "Don't you dare touch her!" and then flung her to the ground. Before I could scold him for being too harsh we were surrounded by over a dozen men yelling and shouting at us.

Another woman, with a baby strapped to her back, swooped in and pulled the woman out of the way just as pistols were being cocked and arrows were being notched. My hands twitched for my own bow, but I made fists and fought the urge. The boys didn't resist the way I did and immediately raised their pistols and aimed right back at the hostile group surrounding us. I heard the chief and Kiyahe come running out of the lodge at the commotion. The chief barked out a command and one of the men responded, I guessed to tell him what had happened. Kiyahe stared at me and I at him, unable to run to each other for fear of igniting a shootout.

After what felt like ages but was probably only a minute at most, I made my move. I slowly shrugged my bow and sheath of arrows off of my shoulders and tossed them to the side before kneeling in the snow with my hands up in surrender. One of their men grabbed my weapon as I told the twins and Jolon to do the same. I heard Kiyahe groan at our disarming and leaving ourselves so vulnerable, but I couldn't think of any other way to defuse the tension. With my head bowed, I asked Kiyahe to explain to the chief our misunderstanding and that we meant no harm.

"And if you could ask him to please ask his people to stop aiming their weapons at us, that would be great too."

Kiyahe spoke in the chief's language, his voice polite and pleading. The chief made the command and the danger dissipated as the people lowered their weapons, threw ours back to us, and dispersed. I waited a moment longer before grabbing my bow and arrows and slowly standing, the boys following my lead. The chief had already walked back to his lodge and I ran into Kiyahe's arms, the weight of fear only fully leaving me when he caught me in an embrace.

Kiyahe brushed my hair out of my face while Jolon filled him in on what had happened.

"It was a misunderstanding is all," I shook my head. "What did the chief say?

Kiyahe sighed, "You know how I told you that the chief had lost his wife and son in childbirth?"

My eyebrows knitted together in confusion, "Yeah but what does that have to do with me?"

"Tatenga took his wife to a white hospital to have their baby and it was a white female doctor who tended her when she died. You remind him of the doctor and he's prejudiced and still hurting over what happened. I could tell we weren't going to get very far with you doing the talking," Kiyahe explained apologetically.

"Oh…" was all I could think to say. I felt another wave of sympathy for the chief, despite his angry demeanor. For someone to be so angry and so hurt for so long was a terrible way to live.

"So, is he going to ally with us?" I finally asked.

"I think he will, he's spiritual enough to consider our legends and logical enough to see the strength in our numbers. I told him to take his time and pray about it. And to convene with their elders. He promised me an answer by tomorrow."

I nodded, "I think we should go back to the bus until then," I said.

"I agree," Kiyahe and Jolon said together. The twins nodded their agreement as well.

And so, we trudged through the snow back to the bus, the footprints from our hike towards the tribe long covered up by wind and fresh snow. Kiyahe hoped the same would happen to our footprints away from the reservation. But just to be sure, he had the twins and Jolon create false roundabout paths in case anyone unfriendly decided to come looking for us. By the time we reached the bus, the winter sun was beginning to set, and we were all frozen through and through.

Jolon filled Aiyana in on our visit while the twins planned our dinner and Kiyahe did a routine check on the bus and scooped snow out from around the tires. I busied myself hanging everyone's clothes from doorknobs and the backs of chairs so that they could dry.

Everyone ate in contemplative silence that night and there was no after dinner banter or conversation like usual. We were all wondering what decision the Choctaw would come to by the next day and worrying that our previous successes might have made us arrogant in the end of our journey. It was maddening to lie in wait, so we all went to bed early, hoping tomorrow would bring warmth, not just from the weather, but from our last tribe as well.

That night I had a dream that I was fifteen again and laying in my bed at home in Atlantis. It was the middle of the night and I had just woken up, thirsty for a glass of water. I tiptoed down the stairs in the dark when the glow of the fireplace caught my eye and the warmth of it beckoned be closer. I stood in front of it, the heat making me drowsy, and suddenly I had forgotten what I had come downstairs for. The mantle was decorated with stockings and snow globes; it was almost Christmas. The warmth was so pleasant at first, but then, the longer I stood there, the more it became uncomfortable. The heat was making me sweat and my pajamas were sticking to me. My droopy eyelids snapped open when I realized the fire was no longer contained in the fireplace but was spreading along the walls and across the floor towards me. I opened my mouth to scream but no sound came out. I commanded my legs to run but they stood locked in place. Terrified, I watched until the fire was completely surrounding me. Within seconds it was torching its way up my body, scorching, burning. I screamed my soundless scream in agony at the pain. I heard blasts over the roar of the fire but was too trapped in my own pain to wonder where they came from.

The walls and ceilings of my home gave way like a house of cards, only with big crashes instead of papery flutters. A December blizzard whirred around me like a wintry tornado. I prayed that the wind and snow would put out the fire that ensconced me. And it did, after a very slow and agonizing time. When the fire was finally quenched, I fell over in the icy snow, still unable to move or scream for help. The snow covered my blistered skin, at first blissfully numbing me. But then, after a while, the snow started to burn me as well, an icy, razor-like burn. The blizzard burned on as it buried me alive.

I believe much trouble and blood would be saved if we opened our hearts more.
— Chief Joseph, Nez Perce.

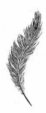

Chapter Fifteen

"Marie! Wake up, Marie!" Kiyahe shouted at me as he shook my shoulders. I lurched up into a sitting position, gasping for air. "It's alright now, you're safe," Kiyahe soothed me. I looked around me for the inferno, but it was quiet, dark, and safe in the bus bedroom. I wiped the back of my hand across my forehead and felt the beads of sweat that had formed in my hairline. My cheeks were wet; I must have been crying while trapped inside my nightmare.

"What happened?" Kiyahe whispered urgently. "What did you see?"

I grimaced as the memory of the fire came flooding back to me. "There was a fire," I whispered hoarsely. My throat felt as if I'd also been screaming in my sleep. "I was at home, in front of the fireplace, and then everything was on fire. *I* was on fire. And then the snow came and the cold was burning me. I just kept burning and burning..." I trailed off.

Even in the dark I could see the protective concern in Kiyahe's eyes. "It's another vision. There's going to be trouble with the Choctaw tomorrow, isn't there? They're going to hurt you."

I didn't want it to be true, but I knew better than to doubt my visions now. All I could do was nod and try to look brave.

"I know I can't convince you to give up on this tribe and leave, so I won't try. But I think everyone needs to come with us tomorrow. You need to have as much protection as possible," Kiyahe said.

He didn't ask me for approval of the idea, but I nodded in agreement anyway. Having all my protectors with me didn't give me solace though. It only made me worry that more people could get hurt along with me.

We laid down again and I let Kiyahe hold me. Neither of us went back to sleep that night.

꩜

I didn't want to tell the others about my vision the next morning. Their excitement about heading home was almost tangible and I didn't want to ruin everyone's good mood only to scare them about something we couldn't control. Kiyahe respected my decision not to tell them but insisted on getting everyone focused, alert, and fully armed before we left for the Choctaw reservation. Thankfully, no one asked why *all* of my protectors were accompanying us that day.

The winds and snows from the night before covered our tracks nicely, which gave me some sense of relief. However, it also forced us to trudge along slowly to the reservation, breaking out a new path through the deep snow. It took us twice as long as the day before to get to the reservation.

When we got there, the tribe was in an uproar. People congregated out in the cold, forming mobs and shouting at each other in their Native language. As soon as we were in the peripherals of the people, my protectors flocked around me, Kiyahe in front of me, the twins at my sides, and Aiyana and Jolon behind my heels. I kept one hand on Kiyahe's back to let him know I was close.

We walked around the outside edge of the shouting mob to get to the chief's lodge, trying to be inconspicuous. "What are they shouting about?" I asked, just loud enough for Kiyahe to hear.

"Gee I wonder," Neka scoffed from my right. I shot a glare at him, catching his eye roll in return. I threw an elbow in his rib at the same time Aiyana stepped on the heel of his shoe.

"Enough," Kiyahe said sternly. "They're divided over the chief's decision to join our alliance."

My heart lifted with pleasant surprise and just a hint of hope, "The chief will join us?" I asked.

"Sounds like it, but about half of the tribe isn't happy about it," Kiyahe answered.

I looked over my shoulder at the protesters with their fists raised in the air, their eyes filled with fury. I shuddered.

When we cut in front of the mob to stop in front of the chief's lodge, the din of the protests died down and everyone watched us.

Kiyahe turned to me, "I have to go in to speak to him, wait out here and don't move an inch away from our group. Promise me?"

I nodded, "I promise." And I meant it. Kiyahe gave me a quick kiss on the cheek before turning and entering the lodge. From within my cocoon of protectors I watched as the protesters stared at me and I stared past them. The silence was awkward, and the tension was threatening.

After what felt like the longest time, Kiyahe and the chief emerged from the lodge and the chief announced in his Native tongue of our newly formed alliance. The people roared with anger and the chief waved his hands to silence them while Kiyahe returned to my side. As the chief spoke, Kiyahe interpreted for me.

"My people!" the chief boomed. "Our visitors have travelled across most of the country to unite our friends and enemies. They do this so that we may rebuild a new nation and stand firm in our homelands. So that our children and our children's children will grow up on the lands their ancestors and the Great Spirit intended for them. So that we may never again have our homes stolen from us."

"She will steal our land!" someone shouted.

"We cannot trust the whites again!" another added.

"My children!" the chief thundered. "I know, better than many, how the whites can be deceiving. But I cannot, and you cannot, live with clouded eyes of hatred. Their chief's son has begged me to clear my own eyes and when I did I realized that the words of these young people," the chief swallowed before glancing quickly at me, "the words of this young woman, are true. If we don't unite we cannot protect our lands. We will perish the way our ancestors did, and our children may not have a place in this new world at all. This is our second chance, given to us from the Great Spirit, and we would be foolish to throw it away over prejudice and hatred!"

There was silence instead of uproar after the chief's speech and I felt tears prick my eyes with hope.

"My people," the chief concluded, "will we protect our land and future generations?"

Some shouted their agreement, others spoke it softly, others merely nodded. In my peripherals though, I saw some walk away defeated, not happy with the alliance but not strong enough in numbers to fight it. Among them was the woman who'd raised her hand to me the day before. She walked away holding hands with a man whom I guessed was her husband. I felt the hairs on my neck stand up when they departed.

With the time for speeches over, the Choctaw chief approached each of us in our group and shook our hands, mine included. I asked Kiyahe to give the chief my condolences for his losses all those years ago and of course to thank the chief as well. Some of the people also approached us to meet and speak with us, but most just went back to their daily lives and the warmth of their lodges. A little over an hour later, we left.

Everyone, except Kiyahe and I, was overjoyed at our most recent alliance and the overall success of our journey. Aiyana and Jolon walked with their linked hands swinging merrily between them and the twins raced and wrestled each other in the snow on our walk back. I couldn't stop thinking about my vision and I guessed Kiyahe was thinking about it too. I got the strange feeling that we weren't safe yet, and knew I wouldn't feel relief until we were on the road, away from our most recent hosts.

We got on the bus, everyone buzzing with excitement except Kiyahe and I who were still focused and on alert. Shilah took the wheel and turned us around on the road so that we were facing west, towards home. As he and Kiyahe discussed the best route to get us to Oklahoma, Neka filled Aiyana and Jolon in on what the Potawatomi reservation and the tribe was like. Hearing him talk about home, about our family, lifted my spirits enough to take my mind off of the Choctaw tribe and settle them on the future. Looking out the window at the snowy, blanketed countryside, I realized that Christmas couldn't be far off. I smiled, thinking about Christmas with my new family after a long and eventful journey. It would be a small respite, a small celebration before I set to work leading our newly united nation.

I dozed on and off for much of the snowy drive until a bump in the road jostled me awake. I looked around me; it was nighttime, Neka was passed out on Shilah's couch, Aiyana and Jolon were quietly playing cards under the overhead light in the booth, Shilah was still driving, and Kiyahe was studying the map from his father in the passenger seat. As I watched my protectors, I became aware of a small noise coming from somewhere in the bus. I listened harder to what sounded like a beeping noise. It was subtle but unmistakable. I looked around me for the source of the noise and saw nothing out of the ordinary. After fifteen minutes of wondering what it was, I felt the hairs on the back of my neck stand on end. I had a flashback of the Choctaw woman and her husband who had stepped out early from the gathering that morning.

"Something's wrong," I said aloud. Aiyana and Jolon put down their cards and looked at me in question. Neka remained asleep on the couch. Shilah turned his head slightly to see me in his peripherals while still keeping his eyes on the road. Kiyahe turned around in his seat.

"What is it?" Kiyahe asked me, his eyes mirroring my concern.

"Beeping…I don't know…like an alarm clock or a timer…" I wondered aloud. The others looked at me in confusion, clearly not hearing it. I had another flashback then, of my nightmare.

"The fire," I whispered. And that's when the panic set in. "FIRE!" I screamed.

The last thing I saw before the explosion was a pair of beautiful turquoise eyes.

Confusion.

Panic.

Pain.

Burning.

One minute we were in the safety of the bus, the next there was a deafening blast as the bus imploded. We were thrown in all directions like weightless rag dolls before we hit the snow packed ground with thuds.

The fire burned brighter and hotter than in my nightmare. It surrounded me like a cocoon and all I could think about was the blistering pain as I burned alive. After what felt like a hellish eternity, my mind thrashed against the pain and I began to see flickers of the disaster back in August. People burning, running, and screaming. The woman I'd nearly hit with my car, who'd rolled around wildly in the neighbor's sprinklers, I saw her again through the flames that danced in front of my eyes.

And then there was green and a cool breeze. The meadow from my dream, after I'd been poisoned. It was beautiful and peaceful. I saw the burning woman from my hometown sitting by the river, she was no longer burning but calm and content. I asked her if I could join her by the water, knowing the quenching river would put out the burning heat, but she shook her head no.

"It's not your time yet," she said simply.

Confused and a little hurt by her rejection, I didn't know what else to do but return to the inferno.

Like in my dream, the swirling snow put out the fire before it could torch the life right out of me. The chill was welcoming, the increasing visibility of the wintry night inviting. But then the snow started to bury me, to form a heavy, wet grave over top of me. I commanded my arms and legs to push the snow away, to dig myself out, but I was immobile.

"Don't worry, Marie, I've got you! It's almost out, I promise!"

Kiyahe? Was that his voice on the other side of the icy grave?

I laid under the heavy, suffocating snow for maybe a minute longer before my copper-skinned, blue-eyed protector pushed the snow away from me and the blistering wind stung my open wounds.

"Kiyahe?" I nearly whispered.

"I'm here, Marie, it's ok. You're going to be ok, do you understand me? Stay with me, now!" he shouted at me.

"The others," I whimpered, my fear for them causing a few tears to roll down my face.

"I know, I'll get them. I had put you out first. I had to make sure you were ok. I'll be right back, you wait here."

"Obviously," I whispered, but Kiyahe was already on his feet and gone.

For the longest time it was just me, my pain, and the starry sky above. My wounds burned to my bones and the December air was merciless. I focused on my breathing and keeping my eyelids open.

Eventually I heard shoes crunching in the snow and felt Kiyahe's warm arms scoop me up. I cringed away from the wind and into Kiyahe's chest.

"Where do we go now?" Aiyana asked, her voice surprisingly close. I looked up just enough to see that she had an arm around Kiyahe's neck, leaning on him for support.

"We have to find shelter," Kiyahe grunted from under my weight and part of Aiyana's.

"Well we better find it fast because I don't know how long we can carry this guy!" Jolon shouted over the howl of the wind. I blinked and looked around to see Jolon and Neka carrying a large and unconscious Shilah between them. Wet tears ran silently down Neka's face and froze on his cheeks.

"We'll go west, keep your eyes open for a group of trees or shrubs or rocks, anything that can help break the wind," Kiyahe commanded.

And with that we shuffled ever so slowly through the blizzard. I caught a glimpse of the bus, which was now nothing more than a mangled, smoldering pile. Pieces of the bus and all our belongings had been flung from the wreckage and were now blazing all around us like miniature beacons in the dark. I reached for my necklace from Mahala and Hiawassee instinctively, glad that at least my favorite possession had been spared. The moonless night and the heavy, whipping flakes of snow made visibility almost impossible once we left the glow of the explosion. I gritted my teeth against the pain and the burning and forced myself not to scream.

Somewhere, sometime in the night, we found a shallow creek with dense trees on either side of the slow-moving water. Kiyahe helped Aiyana sit and laid me down beside her, my head resting gently on her lap. I heard the boys drop, more than lay, Shilah down. While Jolon sat in the dirt panting, Neka started sobbing a heart wrenching sob for his dying twin brother. Aiyana gently pushed my wet hair out of my eyes in an uncharacteristic, motherly way, while we rasped and coughed like chain-smokers. Everyone was covered in soot and snow.

Kiyahe allowed them no more than a chance to catch a breath before telling Jolon and Neka to get up so that the three of them could stack rocks and branches around us to provide some shelter. Jolon pulled himself clumsily to his feet but Neka remained with his head in his hands, wailing inconsolably. Kiyahe grabbed him by the collar of his shirt and yanked him up.

"He's alive now but he'll die if we don't protect him from the wind! We all will!" Kiyahe shouted.

"Stop it!" I shouted back, my voice crackling like kindling as I tried to put out some volume.

Kiyahe must have heard me because he glanced at me before sighing and letting go of Neka's shirt.

"I'm sorry," he apologized. "But I need your help right now, ok?"

Neka nodded and wiped his nose on what was left of his sleeve before the three of them set to work.

"Where the hell are we even at?" I asked Aiyana in a raspy voice after a few minutes.

"Arkansas, I think," she coughed, "Kiyahe said we were close to the Oklahoma border just before we blew the hell up."

"Did he say how far from the reservation we are, then?"

"I think about three hours?" Aiyana answered before a dry cough overtook her.

"Three hours isn't bad," I said.

"Three hours by bus, Kaya. Do you know how long that's going to take on foot?" she sniped. I couldn't bring myself to return her snippety attitude. It meant she was ok enough not to be dying.

"I've grown to like long walks," I coughed out a laugh.

Aiyana chuckled at my bad joke. "You would."

Once the boys had gathered everything in the vicinity and piled it around us in a small, crescent shaped wall, we all huddled inside our small sanctuary. Kiyahe and Aiyana gently moved me so my head was now in Kiyahe's lap. Aiyana slumped against Jolon's shoulder, and Neka kept vigilant watch over his brother and cried less audibly than before.

"We need a fire," I told Kiyahe. My survival instincts were at the ready once again. Although I never imagined I would be traveling cross country on foot again. Especially in the dead of winter.

"I thought of that but everything out there is soaked from the wet snow, I won't be able to get anything to light," Kiyahe told me.

"Then we have to drink water and rest," I said.

We took turns helping each other to the water's edge to get a drink. Jolon suggested we splash some water on Shilah's face and when we did, he came to. We kept Shilah talking as long as we could, worried that he had a concussion. Eventually though, we all passed out from exhaustion and pain.

⁂

We were a slow moving and dispirited group the next day. Neka was able to wake Shilah the next morning but we discovered he had broken something in his leg. He hobbled between Neka and Jolon, leaning heavily on them for support. On Jolon's other side, Aiyana clung to him for support as well. I was too badly burned along my arms, torso, and legs to walk, so Kiyahe carried me in his arms.

Kiyahe knew we were close to missing the three-month deadline, if we hadn't already, and that his father would send men out to find us soon. Luckily for us, they would travel the reverse of our journey so, with patience and prayer, we hoped to run into them soon enough. And if they drove, we could ride back home with them and be tended to by a healer quickly.

However, we were like ants in a vast stretch of land and if we missed each other, we would have to walk the whole way home. Shilah and myself were the worst off and I worried that we wouldn't survive the journey, especially with the nights as freezing cold as they were and with all our food and water having to be gathered along the way.

By evening, after walking only a few pitiful miles, we stopped to set up camp just before dark. Kiyahe shot a few rabbits with his grandfather's pistol, the only weapon to survive the explosion, while Jolon, Neka, and Aiyana set up another shelter. Shilah and I were too weak to be of any use. There were just enough dry sticks and branches lying around to build a small fire and cook our small meal.

We continued like that for the next couple days, barely sustaining, slowly healing, steadily moving. But even so, survival in the wilderness, day after day, in the middle of winter, was taking its toll on Aiyana, Jolon, and the twins. Kiyahe and I were faring slightly better, given our past experiences. On the third night, with everyone else exhausted and asleep, Kiyahe and I stayed up a little later than the others, sitting around the luxury of our first decent fire. Despite my hellish inferno experience, I welcomed the fire after several days of walking in the blistering, icy wind.

"Why do you call me Marie?" I asked him as I watched the flickering orange flames. The question had crossed my mind multiple times, but I had never taken the time to ask it. It seemed so trivial given everything that had been going on.

Kiyahe smiled, his familiar sarcasm an even warmer welcome than the fire, "That's your name, isn't it?"

I smiled back, "Yes, but no one calls me by it anymore. Everyone calls me Kaya. Except you."

"Would you rather I called you Kaya?"

"No," I answered, "I mean, I don't really care either way. I just wondered why."

Kiyahe took a deep breath before responding. I watched the white plumes of warm air escape his nostrils when he did. "Well a small part of it is because that's how you introduced yourself when we met, so it's a force of habit I guess."

"But?" I asked.

"But," he continued, "I think the bigger reason is because as annoyingly curious and stubbornly infuriating as that girl that I met was," he chuckled, "and still is… that's the girl I fell in love with. I love you for who you are and not just for who you've become."

"I see," I whispered, a warmth unrelated to the fire spreading inside me.

"I've always kind of wondered though," Kiyahe added, "If you like the name Kaya better or less than Marie? Does it ever make you sad? Like your old name, your old self has died in a way? Or does it feel right? Like Kaya is who you've been all along, like Kaya is who you were meant to be."

I shook my head, "I'm both," I answered. "I will always be Marie, and I will always be Kaya. Remember when I told you what Sihu said? About God having more to care about then the titles people refer to Him by?"

Kiyahe nodded.

"I guess I kind of feel the same way," I shrugged. "I don't care so much about the name as I do about who I am. And what I have to do"

A crooked smile spread across Kiyahe's face and I struggled to control my heart beat. "You're going to make an amazing leader, Marie. You've been one all along."

I laughed, "Well I don't know if 'amazing' is the right word. But I'm certainly trying my hardest."

"Me too," Kiyahe said. "But by the looks of you," he gestured to my charred, scabbing skin, "I'd say I still have room for improvement."

We laughed and talked into the night. Somewhere in our conversations I fell asleep and dreamt of home. My old home and my new home. My old family and my new family. My old self and my new self.

And I was happy.

We survive, and we do more than just survive. We bond, we care, we fight, we teach, we nurse, we bear, we feed, we earn, we laugh, we love, we hang in there, no matter what.

–Paula Gunn Allen, Laguna Pueblo.

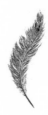

Chapter Sixteen

The sound of a vehicle on the highway woke us early the next morning. I sat up with the others, gritting my teeth against the pain of moving my raw skin. About a half mile away there was a black shape going down the road, a Hummer. Coming from the west, where home was.

Kiyahe was the quickest to react, jumping to his feet and running towards the vehicle, shouting and waving his arms wildly. Neka and Jolon ran after him, also trying to get the Hummer's attention. Aiyana, Shilah, and I stayed behind waiting, hoping we wouldn't have to spend any more time in the frigid countryside.

The driver saw the boys, slowed, and came to a stop just as Kiyahe was reaching the road. Neka and Jolon caught up quickly and our boys' conversation with the driver lasted less than two minutes before they piled in the Hummer, turned off of the road, and came towards us.

It was a group of three men from our tribe. Neka and Shilah's father, Muata, was one of them. Muata's face when he saw his injured son was split between relief and worry. Relief that his son, both of his sons, were alive, but worry over Shilah's condition. The men quickly crammed us in, not having anticipated the need for two extra seats for my joined protectors, and within ten minutes we were speeding towards home.

When we pulled into the reservation, my heart soared with happiness at finally being home again. I struggled to keep my tears at bay as I looked out of the windows at our people, cheering and clapping in celebration.

We had done it.

The reservation looked so different from when I had first arrived several months ago. Then, it was a dilapidated array of tiny homes, shacks, and shelters. Now, many of the downtrodden homes had been repaired and surrounded by newly built ones. Smoke billowed into the air from chimneys and fire pits and several running vehicles were driving in and out of the area. Everyone was quickly gathering to witness our return, all of them bundled in combinations of hand sewn furs and skins as well as modern outdoor winter wear. We drove to where the ceremonial tipi had been, but it was gone. In its place there was a fairly large cabin and, standing in front of it, waiting for us, were Kiyahe's parents, Ahote and Nakoma. My heart was filled with relief and worry. My God, did we have a lot to tell them!

As we piled out of the Hummer, Kiyahe took my hand to help me out and didn't let go as we approached his parents.

A brief flicker of concern crossed their faces before they quickly masked it and embraced all of us in welcome.

"My young ones you have done so well! We are so happy to see you home and safe!" Nakoma smiled happily.

"Yes, you are all wise and strong beyond your years and we couldn't be more proud of you," Ahote told us.

"Great Spirit, you did not come home unscathed I see!" Nakoma gasped as her gaze took in my burned skin. I looked stupidly at my arm, having temporarily forgotten about the pain in the excitement of our homecoming. Shilah nearly buckled under his injured leg at that moment and Nakoma didn't miss it.

"You have to come inside so you can be tended to, we'll talk more later, and we'll celebrate once you're healed," she declared.

"Yes, but first," Ahote stopped her, eagerness and hope filling his weary face, "Tell me simply, did all of the tribes ally with you? Are we a united people?"

I smiled through my returning pain, "Yes."

And it was true, we had letters of promise from every chief of every tribe we had visited that spoke of their joined alliance. Not all had been as thrilled or as convinced in their promise to be our allies, but they had all agreed just the same. I knew I would have to continue relations with all of them as time went on, as well as gain the trust of others I had not yet met. But that was a job for another day. Right now I needed to rest and heal.

Ahote sighed in happy relief and let his wife usher us inside. The chief went to find a few more pairs of hands that were somewhat experienced in healing or medical practices to help his wife tend to us. In the large living room of the cabin, surrounded by the warmth from a roaring fire and several bowls of smoldering incense, we were made to lie down on makeshift stretchers while Nakoma assessed each of us.

Kiyahe, Jolon, and Neka were released almost immediately as they were little more than hungry and tired. Aiyana was told she had a mild concussion and a small ankle sprain but that she was healing quickly. Shilah was much worse, with a broken shin, fractured ankle, severe burning to one arm, and a severe concussion. Nakoma asked everyone who wasn't bed ridden to leave the cabin because Shilah's tibia had begun to set wrong and it needed to be re-broken to set correctly. Kiyahe had refused to leave my side, so he, Aiyana, and I plugged our ears and gritted our teeth to try and drown out Shilah's screams while his leg was re-broken and set properly.

Although I had nothing broken, I had the worst burns and they covered my front and back along my torso, arms, and legs. Luckily my face, head, hands, and feet had escaped the burning. I was stripped and scraped, the pain of which was agonizing. I had to muffle my screams and curses with my pillow as one of the female assistants scraped the dead and infected skin from my body. Then I was washed with an array of liquids to clean my wounds, which made me scream all over again because it felt as if they were wiping me down with acids. Finally, they slathered me with a cream that soothed and cooled me before they bandaged me like a mummy. Kiyahe held my hand through it all.

While Ahote spread the word that we had succeeded in our journey, he also told our people that we would not celebrate until our group was fully healed and ready to tell our story. Of course, our arriving home, broken and burned, sparked question and controversy within the tribe. If we had made friends and spread peace along our journey, why were we in such terrible shape? How had we received our injuries? Ahote did his best to placate the tribe and promised that all would be explained when Kaya and her protectors were healed.

Nakoma insisted that we rest as much as possible and allowed very few visitors besides my small group of uninjured protectors.

Muata was our first visitor and spent most of his time sitting with Neka at Shilah's bedside, the three of them talking quietly. Every time he came though, he made the effort to say hello and ask Aiyana and I how we were doing.

Mahala was our next visitor and her and I broke down into tears immediately upon seeing each other. Although she still refused to speak, she held my hand tightly and listened to me tell her how I had gotten hurt and how much I had missed her and Hiawassee while I was gone. I had worn the necklace she'd made me throughout the entire trip, never once taking it off. As she was leaving, I asked her to bring Hiawassee to see me soon and she nodded with a smile.

Hiawassee, her daughter, was our third visitor. The little girl I had first met and spent precious little time with had changed in the months since I'd last seen her. She was slightly taller and leaner, her cheeks not as full with baby fat now. Her raven black hair hung even lower and thicker. Her eyes seemed wiser, more like her mother's. But her heartwarming smile had remained the same and it lit up the room just like it had before. When she saw me, she flew across the room like a little bird and flung her arms around me like I was her favorite person in the world. I yelped slightly in pain but quickly covered it with a smile just as her mother tapped her shoulder with a stern finger and showed her how to be gentle with me. Her naïve and youthful joy made the whole room smile and her lightheartedness lingered even after she'd left.

A couple weeks after we'd returned home, Aiyana started vomiting. At first, we were alarmed, worried that someone had made another attempt to poison us, but Aiyana admitted she had been feeling nauseous for some time and blew it off as a stomach bug. Shilah, slowly returning to his old teasing self every day, joked that it was probably one of the gross teas Nakoma was making us drink. I wasn't sure what to think but I watched Aiyana closely as her vomiting continued.

A few nights later I had a dream that I was holding a beautiful baby boy, swaddled in furs. He was awake; smiling, squirming, and gurgling as happy babies do. One of his little bronze fists was gripping my finger and the other was curled around a small, onyx colored arrowhead. His smile was bright and unabashed, almost jovial. A small tuft of beautiful black hair, the weight of feathers, covered the top of his head. And a pair of onyx colored eyes, the same shade as the arrowhead that he clung to, peeked up at me. Those eyes seemed wise and almost critical as they looked back at me. Like the boy thought that *I* was the silly, infantile one.

He was familiar to me in a way that I couldn't quite place. I had seen numerous Native babies along our journey, but I knew this one wasn't one of them. Still, I had seen those features before, those bemused eyes, and that carefree smile. A dozen memories flashed across my mind, trying to place where I had seen him before. But all I could focus on in my memories were the faces of my protectors. My eyes lingered on the arrowhead in the baby's hand for a long time before I realized who he was. Who his parents were.

♫

What seemed a beautiful and exciting revelation to me didn't seem so to Aiyana.

When I suggested the idea that she might be having morning sickness because she might be pregnant, she looked at me for a very long time before exploding loud enough that anyone outside the cabin would surely have heard her loud and clear.

"That isn't possible! I haven't…only once…we…NO! It's a stomach bug, Kaya. That's it, end of story!"

"You have to admit it's possible, Aiyana!" I shouted back at her. "That night in the bus after we gained the Creek as allies, remember?"

"This is so gross; I *so* don't want to hear this conversation!" Shilah moaned from his stretcher between Aiyana and I.

"You're wrong, Kaya! Get the idea out of your head because that's not what's wrong with me," Aiyana huffed, crossing her arms in defiance.

"There's nothing *wrong* about it!" I said, exasperated. "You're in love, you care about each other, you have a home here and people who will support you, what are you so worried about?!"

Nakoma came in then, with the morning bucket of snow to boil into water. She took one look at the three of us and knew something was up. Aiyana and I turned to look at each other.

"Don't you dare!" she hissed through her teeth.

I turned back to Nakoma defiantly. "Aiyana's pregnant," I said clearly. Air whistled through Aiyana's teeth in anger, but she held her tongue, she had enough respect for Nakoma not to cuss me out in front of her.

Nakoma looked at Aiyana and I could see her eyes reassessing the sick Sioux girl.

"How long?" Nakoma asked her.

Aiyana's nostrils flared and after a few moments it was clear that she would not entertain the idea in the slightest. I answered for her, "A little over three weeks."

Nakoma shook her head, "Three weeks is rather early to be having morning sickness."

"I know she's pregnant," I said unwaveringly.

Nakoma turned her eyes on me then, "How can you be sure, dear?"

I swallowed, "I…I dreamt it. I know it's true." Dear God, I thought. The truth of my visions was not a conversation I wanted to have right now! This was supposed to be about Aiyana!

Nakoma and I stared at each other. And my unsaid words, my explanation for how I *knew,* was plastered on my face. But I was too cowardly to talk about it yet. I tried to turn the shaman's attention back to the more pressing issue. "Surely we could find a pregnancy test, right? To prove it?" I asked.

Nakoma tore her eyes from me and returned to the previous issue, but I knew the topic of my visions wouldn't be put off for long. "Yes, I'm sure we have some somewhere."

Aiyana didn't talk to me after that. Her silent treatment hurt me at first but by the next day I had convinced myself that I was doing the right thing and that she would come around eventually. Aiyana's medical treatment and diet were changed after that, and a few days later when she missed her cycle, Nakoma had her take the test and she was indeed, pregnant. I congratulated her, but she ignored me. When I asked her if she was going to tell Jolon, she only glared at me. I threatened to tell him myself but secretly I knew that I wouldn't do that to Aiyana. Jolon deserved to know the truth but it wasn't my business to tell him and he would find out soon enough, even if Aiyana procrastinated about it.

The day of Christmas Eve, Nakoma released us so that we could enjoy the festivities and tell about our journey to our impatient tribe. Aiyana was fully recovered but Shilah had to walk with a cast and crutches and both of us were instructed to come back once a day to have our burns cleaned and bandages changed. Kiyahe, Neka, and Jolon had been staying with Muata while we healed and now Shilah would join them and Kiyahe would return to his parent's cabin. Aiyana and I would stay with Mahala and Hiawassee. The separation at night from Kiyahe had been, and would continue to be, strange and lonely. But it was bearable as long as I had some of my new family to stay with.

The Christmas Eve celebration was glowing and festive. Everyone decorated their homes and dressed up for the evening. We gathered in a newly built gathering lodge at one end of the reservation. Kiyahe had informed me that our tribes numbers had grown as a few dozen nomads had settled with the Potawatomi in our absence.

Our group rejoined just in time to enter the gathering lodge together, Kiyahe and I holding hands in the front, Aiyana and Jolon behind us, the twins behind them, and Muata, Mahala, and Hiawassee trailing us. Everyone inside yipped and cheered when we entered.

Our tribe had been very busy while we were gone. Aside from adopting new members and building new homes and gathering places, they had also re-established electricity in the public buildings. The large gathering lodge glowed brightly as bulbs whirred overhead and a cozy heat filled the room and chased away the cold that slipped in every time the door was opened. Ours was the second tribe I'd seen accomplish this feat, but I knew the others wouldn't be far behind.

Decorations adorned every wall and corner of the massive main room and a ten-foot Christmas tree, that had been pushed to the side to make room for tables and chairs, stretched towards the high rafters of the ceiling. Little hand sewn moccasins, feathers, dreamcatchers, and strings of beads and berries hung from the branches along with a few store-bought ornaments from before the disaster. The topper was a Native angel with wings and a colorful woven star behind her.

Several tables had been pushed together to make a new, very long, head table that would satisfy the seating needed for our large group. The chief and I sat in the middle of the table with Nakoma at his side and Kiyahe at mine, followed by the rest of our group. Before serving our group himself, Ahote said a special prayer, thanking the

Great Spirit for our safe and successful return. Besides the tender, well marinated elk roast and fresh, hot fry bread, I wasn't exactly sure what all was on my plate, but everything tasted amazing and I ate without question. Everyone ate in silence at our table while the buzz of chatter filled the room from the rest of the tribe.

When most of the tribe had finished their food, and a few were going back for seconds, Ahote stood and announced that I would share the story of our journey across the country. I hesitated, there was so much to tell! How could I keep it all straight?! Kiyahe squeezed my hand in encouragement under the table and I gulped rather audibly before I stood and recounted our journey to my people.

Occasionally I had to turn to Kiyahe and the rest of my group to help me keep everything straight and, after a while, they joined in as active participants in the regaling, which helped me feel more comfortable. Everyone had something to add to the story. Kiyahe complimented me often, saying that I had a talent for negotiating with the other tribes and for remaining levelheaded and strong. Aiyana and Jolon shed additional light on their own tribes' measurement of me. And the twins gave humorous commentary that would get our tribe laughing or smiling, lightening the mood. I stuck to the facts and occasionally complimented my protectors for being as valiant as they were encouraging.

When I talked about my visions, jaws fell open and I could feel Nakoma and Ahote's eyes boring into me. I kept talking and kept my head up in front of my tribe, but I couldn't keep my voice from quieting a decibel and my palms from beginning to sweat. Kiyahe reached for my hand, where everyone, including his parents could see it, and grasped it firmly, trying to communicate his support. I didn't connect the dots for the people about what my being a shaman meant and I didn't have to. Hushed whispers spread like wildfire and I tried to keep the blush off of my face. If I wasn't entirely convinced that I was indeed, a shaman, I would never have dared bring it up. But I was convinced. I knew what I was. Who I was.

As I'd guessed, Ahote and Nakoma did not bring up my shaman claims in front of the tribe. They would talk with me alone, after the dinner, and I would be honest with them. When we finished telling our story, Ahote said another prayer and a boisterous celebration began. Sure enough, Nakoma approached me as our table was being cleared.

"I think we have more to talk about, why don't we step in the next room?" she suggested.

I nodded and let her escort me out of the main room, Ahote and Kiyahe following behind us.

The adjacent room was set up like a conference room, a large, hand carved wooden table at the center, surrounded by folding chairs. Outside the window, soft snow flurries blew wildly. We all sat at one end of the table.

"Kaya, dear girl," Nakoma started, "You told us when you came here that you were having dreams, *visions*, that led you here."

I nodded even though it wasn't a question.

"And we believed you fully, obviously you were, *are*, Kaya. But we had thought the visions had stopped once you learned the truth about yourself. That they were only for the purpose of leading you here. But you say you have had them even since then?" Nakoma asked.

"Yes," I answered her slowly. "They don't come every night, just…just when I need them. When He wants to warn me or prepare me for something."

"He being the Great Spirit?" she asked.

"Yes," I said. "The Hopi shaman suggested the idea to me, but I didn't, *couldn't*, believe it. Not until He spoke to me and showed me my parents. And then I knew… I know."

Nakoma leaned back in her chair, as if my answers had exhausted her. She studied me while her husband took over the conversation.

"The legend never said Kaya was a shaman, but it didn't say she *couldn't* be either. If this is true, and you are the next shaman of our tribe, that means you will live among the Potawatomi here, leading us, as well as leading the other tribes that you've united," Ahote said.

"It looks like we just established our new capitol then," Kiyahe mused. His parents nodded in silent agreement.

"And," Ahote continued, "If you are the next shaman then that means that you and Kiyahe will marry and take mine and my wife's places someday."

Kiyahe and I looked at each other and I lost myself in his eyes for the millionth time. My protector. My chief. My love. My *husband.*

Kiyahe's mouth twitched with the threat of a smile before he recovered and spoke seriously to his parents. "I wouldn't want anyone else beside me. I love her."

"I love him too," I said, trying to convey the truth of it with my eyes to his parents. "I know you didn't like the idea of it before. I know I'm not good enough for him and I don't deserve him. And that I was meant to be Kaya. But I think I'm also meant to love him." I looked to my protector then, "We're meant to love each other," I smiled.

Nakoma laughed a short laugh and when I looked at her, her eyes were glistening with unshed tears. "My dear girl, it was never that we thought you weren't good enough or not deserving of our son! We couldn't ask for anyone better! We only worried that love would distract you from uniting the tribes. And obviously it did nothing but strengthen your ties with them and each other. You will be our shaman, Kaya." She laughed again, "And my future daughter!"

"That is if you will have each other," Ahote smiled.

"Always," Kiyahe said devotedly.

"Always," I repeated through my own happy tears.

Love is something you and I must have. We must have it because our spirit feeds upon it. We must have it because, without it, we become weak and faint. Without love, our self-esteem weakens. Without it, our courage fails. Without love, we can no longer look out confidently at the world. With love, we are creative. With love, we march tirelessly. With love, and with love alone, we are able to sacrifice for others.

–Chief Dan George, Salish.

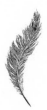

Chapter Seventeen

Ahote and Nakoma returned to the party then, giving us a few minutes of privacy. I let Kiyahe pull me into his arms and kiss me, openly and passionately. The few times we broke our kisses we were laughing and smiling. There were no words to express our joy. All the months of worrying and hiding our affections were over.

When the warmth of our embrace started to climb to a dangerous temperature, I worried about someone coming to look for us. I reluctantly broke out of Kiyahe's grasp and suggested that we return to the party. He agreed even though his eyes, and I feared mine as well, communicated that that's the last place we wanted to be at that moment.

We eased into the crowd in the main room where the party was in full swing. The twins were dancing with some very pretty nomad girls on the makeshift dance floor and Jolon and Aiyana were sitting in chairs along the wall. Jolon's usual boyish excitement was buried deep under an intense look of fear and worry. His eyes refused to leave Aiyana's as she stared intently at the floor.

"Keep the twins out of trouble, will you? I'm going to sit with Aiyana for a moment," I told Kiyahe. His eyes moved to the not-so-happy couple by the wall and he nodded before slipping in amongst the dancers to join the twins.

My first concern was that Aiyana had finally told Jolon the truth about her condition and that he was not happy about becoming a father. But when I reached them and asked what was wrong, Aiyana shot me a warning glare while Jolon explained.

"She got sick a few minutes ago and doesn't feel well," Jolon explained, apparently still oblivious to his girlfriend's pregnancy.

"Why don't you go get a cool rag for her head and I'll sit with her for a while?" I suggested.

He didn't have to be asked twice, Jolon jumped up and left, eager to be of help to his love. I sat down next to Aiyana who was still giving me the silent treatment.

"If you want to ignore me like we're in the third grade then go ahead. I'll talk, and you can listen," I threw at her. From watching her and the twins, I knew Aiyana was best provoked when someone threw her own attitude back at her.

"I think it's a wonderful thing that you're gonna have a baby. Jolon seems like he would be a great father and you have a new tribe who loves you and will take care of you and the baby like you were their own," I told her.

I got an eye roll out of her, but no commentary.

"Do you want to know the gender?" I asked.

"I don't care what the gender is…I just…I just hope it's healthy," Aiyana finally mumbled.

"Why wouldn't it be healthy? You and Jolon are in great shape."

"My mother," Aiyana all but whispered.

My mouth snapped shut with understanding then. Her mother was mentally ill, stricken with severe schizophrenia. The illness had brought her to the point where she couldn't take care of herself and had to have others watch and care for her constantly. Aiyana never talked about all she'd seen and experienced with her mother's condition. But she had mentioned to me before how she hoped she would never become like her mother. And now she feared that her child ran the risk of becoming like his grandmother.

"Aiyana," I said softly, taking her hand in mine. Aiyana wasn't usually a touchy-feely person, but she was so distraught with worry that she didn't pull away from me. "You're gonna have a healthy baby. I know it, I *feel* it. And even if that weren't true, we would all love it just the same. You love your mother, despite her challenges. We would love you and your baby too. But I'm telling you, you have nothing to worry about. The baby I saw in my dream was absolutely perfect."

Aiyana chewed on what I said for a minute before finally nodding and lifting her head to look at me. "I wouldn't believe it if I hadn't already seen how right you always are. That gets kind of annoying you know? You always being right."

I smiled, "Trust me, it can be annoying on my end, too."

Aiyana sighed, "I suppose I need to tell Jolon then, huh?"

"Yes," I answered, "He deserves to know. And I'm sure he'll be thrilled."

"Well then," Aiyana said as she stood and smoothed out her ornately beaded dress, "I better go find my baby daddy."

I laughed as she melted into the crowd to tell her lover something much more important than to forget about the cold rag.

My own love came to me then, gently pulling me from my chair to the dance floor.

"What was that about?" he asked, his smile exuberant and contagious.

I smiled back, "Just some feminine bonding and encouragement, you wouldn't be interested."

"I'm interested in anything that concerns my future wife," Kiyahe drawled in my ear as he moved me to Vance Joy's, "Fire and the Flood."

I blushed heavily at the word 'wife', "That's going to take some getting used to."

"Would a ring help it feel more real?" Kiyahe asked.

My breath caught in my throat as he pulled a delicate, sparkling ring out of his pocket. The band was white gold, pure and perfect. The center stone was a turquoise the exact shade of his eyes. For the dozenth time that evening, my eyes pricked with tears.

"I've had it since we were in Nebraska with the Pawnee," he explained. "I was out scouting and it was in a pile of rubble, right on top. Like it was waiting for me. So I picked it up and it was like it was designed exactly for you. It was perfect."

He slid it onto my finger where it nestled between the knuckles on my left ring finger. He was right, it *was* perfect.

"Do you like it?" he asked, a faint hint of nervousness in his voice.

"I love it and I love you," I said.

He moved me in small circles around the lodge floor and we hummed the rest of the song together.

"I have one more surprise for you," Kiyahe said when the song had ended, his voice low and sultry. The electricity in it and the curiosity over what else he could possibly have for me gave me new energy. I let him unwrap my porcelain arms from around his tawny neck and lead me by the hand. We went to the front door where we had left our winter coats hanging on pegs on the wall.

"Where are we going?" I asked.

"I said it was a surprise, didn't I?" he teased.

"Is it far? Will we come back to the party?" How long will we be gone?" I fired the questions at him, my curiosity claiming my mouth.

"Do you EVER stop asking questions?!" Kiyahe laughed loudly as we walked out into the Christmas snow.

I rolled my eyes at him and continued asking questions which he continued to ignore. Finally, we made it across the reservation to a road on the outskirts. I didn't realize what the surprise was until we were right up to it.

A bus.

A tour bus like the one we'd nearly been blown to pieces in.

"You got me a bus?" I asked dubiously.

Kiyahe turned to me, his smile huge. "Yeah I did. Well, some guys from the tribe did. They've been repairing all sorts of vehicles and this is to replace ours for when we go on more trips to visit more tribes."

I stared at him like he'd lost his mind, what kind of a gift was a bus?

"Come on, you'll like it!" he nearly shouted, pulling my arm to make me follow. "It's much nicer than the one we had before."

Kiyahe continued droning on about the bus as we came up the steps, shook off the snow, and slipped off our coats.

"Here, let me start it so we can get some heat going in here," he said. When he did, the engine purred like a wild cat instead of chugging and sputtering like our old bus did.

I fidgeted with my ring, as Kiyahe started giving me the tour. The bus, although it was laid out the same, really *was* much nicer. And as the heat filled in the spaces and Kiyahe showed me how the lights dimmed, it became almost romantic. I started feeling happy and a little sleepy.

When we got to the bedroom, Kiyahe suddenly ran out of things to say. I smiled at the idea of what might be going through his head. How do you brag about how comfortable the bed is without seeming like you're hinting at something? The soft notes from the stereo filled the silence. It was another Vance Joy song- "Georgia." A slow love song.

"We should probably go back now," Kiyahe said, his voice crackling like a low-lit fire.

"We should," I agreed softly.

We didn't move though. We stood there staring at anything but the bed or each other.

Finally, Kiyahe took a deep breath and gently took my hand to lead me out. But the minute we touched I felt that electric shock again. Felt the warmth that spread from my head to my fingertips to my toes. I wondered if maybe he felt it too because he didn't try to pull me out. He just stood there, looking at my ring standing out from our hands. The warmth turned to a blazing heat and I knew we wouldn't be leaving the bus anytime soon.

❧

Laying there in the smooth sheets, lovingly and intimately tangled. That would always be my happiest memory.

Of course there were things to worry about. Would someone come looking for us? Would someone find us? What would everyone say if they knew. What would Kiyahe's parents think? What were the chances we were now in the same situation as Aiyana and Jolon?

But I was so content and so blissfully happy that the worries were no more than harmless flies. Less than that, they couldn't even touch me.

Kiyahe was right, this was a wonderful gift.

I watched my protector sleep as the dawn began to paint the horizon outside our window. When he finally woke, we smiled at each other like guilty high school kids. The memory of the night before was so strong that I found myself pressing against Kiyahe again, wanting to add to it.

Not wanting it to end. He had to be slower and gentler the second time, we were both new at love making and the first time had left me sore in places I had never been before.

When the morning light had broken across the horizon, we regretfully had to untangle from each other and re-dress. Kiyahe worried about whether his mother would find out and, if she did, whether she would forbid us from seeing each other until our vows were spoken. I was grateful for my silent guardian, Mahala, who wouldn't scold me or tell anyone, even if she wanted to.

Of course, my new roommate, Aiyana, would slap me stupid if she found out that I had done the exact thing that had caused her current condition. Although she was warming to the idea, it wasn't exactly what she'd had planned nine months from now.

We agreed to keep it to ourselves and tell no one, not even my other protectors. If word got back to Kiyahe's mother and she kept us from seeing each other. It would be absolute torture for us.

We also agreed not to sleep together again until after we were married. Although it would be hard, it would give us something to look forward to.

We walked through a quiet, still sleeping reservation that Christmas morning. The sky was a beautiful pale pink and before long, the sun would shine on the glistening snow. For that day anyways, the clouds would be absent. Kiyahe walked me to Mahala's and kissed me goodbye before jogging off towards his parent's cabin. I slipped inside, quiet as a mouse.

Mahala and Hiawassee were still asleep on the newly built queen size bed they shared. Aiyana's twin size bed was empty.

"Stayed up a little late, did we?" she whispered. I jumped in surprise but clamped a hand over my mouth to keep from making any noise. Aiyana's voice was every bit the concerned mother, but her eyes shined with mischief. It was under those sharp eyes though, that I noticed dark circles.

"How long have you been up?" I asked in a hushed whisper.

She shrugged, "Just a few minutes really. I got sick again."

"Do you want some coffee?" I offered. As much as I hated the foul-tasting stuff, I was still rather tired myself.

"I suppose," she yawned, "The other two have been stirring so I'm sure they'll be up soon."

Aiyana surprisingly didn't badger me with questions while I searched for coffee and a percolator. I supposed, though, that the truth of my late-night outing was written all over my face and she didn't need to ask. Once I got the water boiling in the percolator, Aiyana flung a small package across the table towards me.

"What's this?" I asked.

"I know your dense head is filled with Kiyahe right now, but you *do* know it's Christmas, right?" she sniped. "It's for you."

I added the coffee before joining her at the table, slowly unwrapping the small newspaper parcel. Inside were three little ceramic figurines. A Native woman, a man, and a little baby. They were clothed in colorful scraps of cotton and bundled in a little drawstring bag.

"Hiawassee wanted to make you something for Christmas, so we stayed up late making little crafts. Turns out I suck at weaving and sewing and pretty much everything else. Mahala showed me how to shape the clay and bake it in the wood stove. And Hiawassee helped me paint and dress them," she explained.

"Your little family," I smiled.

Aiyana smiled a small smile back, "They have magnets inside them, so you can connect them. And the little bag is so you can take them with you."

"I love them. I wish I had made everyone else gifts too," I said sadly.

"You've given us so much more Kaya," said a woman's voice behind me. I turned to see that Mahala had woken and come up behind me. I struggled to close my mouth at the sound of her voice. I had always imagined that it would sound brash and harsh, in the way her face was often set, and her demeanor was. But instead it was warm and motherly.

Aiyana, apparently unaware of Mahala's silent reputation, recalled my attention. "I won't be able to travel with you for a while. It's too dangerous…in my condition," she said. "So, I thought you could take us with you."

I nodded, "I will. And I'll miss you."

Aiyana rolled her eyes, "Don't get all sappy on me now, pour us some coffee already."

And our morning continued. Mahala returned to her silence, although I was happy to know that she was beginning to share her voice. Perhaps she would come out of her long depression and resume speaking. And then perhaps Hiawassee would follow suit.

Mahala and Hiawassee had made me a bracelet to match the necklace they'd given me before my second journey. Wearing my necklace, new bracelet, and the ring from Kiyahe, I felt almost like I was decked in royal jewels.

The people of the tribe gifted each other with an array of handmade gifts and salvaged gifts from the disaster. Hiawassee was thrilled to have a slightly used baby doll and a hand sewn, beaded dress from her mother. Aiyana had made more ceramic figurines of everyone in our household for Hiawassee to play with. And I gave her another of my necklaces from my old life. Mahala gave Aiyana lots of maternity clothes and a pair of extra cushioned, handmade moccasins. The four of us ate breakfast around the table, enjoying the beautiful Christmas morning.

Kiyahe came by shortly after. When I answered the door, he gently embraced me and kissed me softly. The electricity from his touch was overwhelmingly distracting. He and I spent a little more time at Mahala's before going to Muata's where Jolon and the twins were working on an old Chevy pickup that was Muata's gift to his sons. Jolon was on cloud nine, talking animatedly and smiling nonstop. It was apparent that he was thrilled at the idea of becoming a father. He told us he and several other men were going to build a new house for his someday wife and child.

We stayed at Muata's for a little over an hour before Jolon slipped away to visit Aiyana, and Kiyahe and I left to see his parents. Kiyahe assured me his parents had been asleep when he'd gotten home and were oblivious to our activities after the Christmas Eve party. I was still nervous when I walked into their cabin, though. They were both incredibly intuitive people.

But Nakoma embraced me warmly and Ahote behaved as he normally did. If they had suspicions about our late-night activities, they hid them well.

Kiyahe and I ate lunch with his parents, talking and laughing in between bites. At one point, Ahote tried to launch into all the upcoming things I would have to do as a leader of the people but Nakoma hushed him.

"It's Christmas my husband, Kaya has earned a break and we can worry about the rest after the new year," she insisted. Ahote sighed but didn't push it.

That night there was another celebration to end the Christmas holiday and everyone was exuberant during the festivities. Although I'd already accepted Kiyahe's private proposal, he dropped to his knee in front of the entire tribe and proposed to me again in public. I accepted, of course, and the people erupted in cheers. Word had, indeed, spread like wildfire of my being accepted as the next shaman. And the tribe that had been leery of me almost four months ago was now embracing me as a very central part of their own family.

It was the perfect ending to a year that had changed my life so completely.

Young people are the pioneers of new ways. Since they face too many temptations, it will not be easy to know what is best.

–Chief Dan George, Salish.

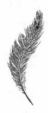

Chapter Eighteen

Life was peaceful and pleasant when we entered the new year. Year one, as everyone was calling it. It seemed fiting as we'd survived such a devastating disaster and were indeed, starting over in so many ways.

Since there was still no internet, phone service, or postal carriers, tribes from all over had begun sending messenger boys, from the ages of fifteen to eighteen, to and from each other to communicate. And with the constant repair of vehicles and roads, the messenger boys were able to travel faster all the time. Communication wasn't as instantaneous as before the Fire Rains, but it was the best we could do.

It was when one of our own messenger boys returned, a young one who'd just turned fifteen, that our brief, happy holiday came to an abrupt halt.

The boy came flying down the main reservation road in a jeep, slush and mud flying out behind his tires. A toddler who was playing too close to the road was quickly snatched by his mother so he wouldn't get hit. Kiyahe and I had just come back from a walk when we saw the boy slam on the breaks and the jeep slide in the gravel in its attempt to stop. Kiyahe defensively pushed me behind him and I had to stand on tip toes to see above his shoulder.

"WAR!" the boy screamed, his pubescent voice cracking as his voice rose to a shrill pitch. "War has started! They're coming for Kaya. They're gonna kill her, they're gonna kill each other, they're gonna kill us all!"

Kiyahe stormed towards the boy and I followed, keeping a hand on his back to let him know I was there. When Kiyahe reached him, he grabbed him roughly by the upper arm and hissed at him. "Quiet Ashkii! You're scaring everyone!"

"Gently, Kiyahe," I said softly. Seeing Kiyahe so intense and angry reminded me of when he'd grabbed Neka after our bus exploded and we were stranded. Kiyahe only lost control when our safety was in danger. When *my* safety was in danger.

The boy, Ashkii, gulped and struggled to regain his breath after all his shouting. He looked at me, too afraid to address Kiyahe, and tried to find some comfort in my eyes when he spoke. "Ahote sent me west, to the Miwok in California. He was worried about the old chief there and your fear of Kalona," he panted.

The mention of Kalona's name gave me chills and Kiyahe bristled in front of me, I thought I might've even heard a growl in his throat.

"And?" I asked, my voice small.

"The old chief is dead. Some said it was only a matter of time, that he was weak and sickly. But the couple who took me in while I was there said they thought Kalona killed him. They don't know how, there wasn't a mark on the chief. But they could feel something was wrong. The chief had made an announcement shortly after you left that Kalona would not become the next chief, that his hostility towards you was intolerable and a risk for the entire tribe. He said he would name a successor in the coming weeks. But he died before one could be chosen," Ashkii explained.

"Oh God," I gasped. My heart sank into what felt like a bottomless hole in my chest. I struggled to find it, to pull it back out. But I was too stunned to think. My past with Kalona may have resulted in the murder of a respected chief. No one could prove it, but I knew it was true. Kalona was not above killing to get what he wanted.

"There's more," Ashkii continued. "Kalona was sending messenger boys out left and right. And elders from the Crow and Blackfoot visited. I overheard them talking about a battle and how many men they could spare. And then a woman came from the Navajo, I heard Kalona and the Navajo woman say they were ready and that more were planning to join them."

My mind raced back to the Crow and Blackfoot tribes, neither of which were my biggest fans. And the Navajo woman, I had the feeling she was the nomadic chief's daughter we'd met. She had expressed her feelings against us when we'd first met but she didn't go against her father's agreement to join us. Apparently, she'd decided an alliance with us was unacceptable.

"They…they want you dead, Kaya," Ashkii whispered. "Kalona especially."

Everyone stood in silence then. Ashkii, Kiyahe and me. Even the onlookers who had heard no more than what the messenger boy had screamed when he'd arrived. I looked out at them and they looked at me. Their expressions twisted with confusion and worry.

I couldn't fake a smile for them, but I could at least try to look brave. I squared my jaw and spoke in a business tone to Ashkii, just loud enough so the closest onlookers could hear and spread my words.

"We can't assume anything. You need to come with us now and share your information with the chief. We have to pray and decide what to do," I said, trying to keep my voice even.

Both boys nodded and the three of us went back to Ahote's cabin to share the terrible news. My heart and my stomach had disappeared into the black hole inside me when Ashkii repeated everything to Ahote and Nakoma. It sounded worse the second time. I felt like I was drowning.

We'd come back home, thinking ourselves successful when we were anything but.

My purpose had been to unite the tribes together. To protect ourselves, our land, and our homes for the future generations. To bring peace.

All I'd managed to do was create a division amongst the people. To create a smaller united front…against me.

A dozen well versed and powerful speeches wasn't going to change thousands of people's minds overnight. And signatures on pieces of paper weren't going to prove loyalty. Only action would convince them.

But would my first action be to fight against my own nation? The one I was supposed to peacefully lead?

The only one I could imagine fighting, possibly killing, was Kalona. He had tried to kill me. He had wanted me dead. He had started this uprising against me. But he was so strong and already appeared to have many in support of him.

My thoughts turned to my protectors then. Aiyana wouldn't have to stand with me, her condition would keep her safe and well out of harm's way. But what about Jolon? Would he be expected to protect me, or would he be allowed to stay with his pregnant girlfriend? Then there were the twins, one of whom was still recovering from his injuries...

And then there was my soul-bound, life-long protector. Kiyahe would fight to the death for me. Not just because he was bound to, but because he loved me.

And I couldn't bring myself to let him.

I couldn't let the fight, let my enemies, come here. It would risk too many lives that I loved.

I had to slip away, alone, and go to them. I had to stop the fighting before it started. Not only for my tribe, my family, my protectors, and my love. But for the future. I had to find a way to stop this without losing anyone, including myself. The legend clearly said that if I failed to unite the people, they would perish. They *had* to learn to unite and I *had* to be the one to teach them.

Ahote broke through my fear-filled thoughts with musings of his own plan.

"We must wait here for them. If we run, we look like cowards, guilty of something we haven't done. We'll send messenger boys to every tribe Kaya visited, except the ones Ashkii has reported on, and ask them to come here and stand with us. We can't let this break out into a war and we can't let them touch Kaya. I think we should move her. Send her somewhere nearby until it's safe to bring her back and address the masses."

"Gathering numbers might make it look like we're assembling our own army. It could make things worse," Kiyahe strategized.

"Yes, and many leaders won't want to risk the lives of the few people they have left. And if they aren't fully devoted to Kaya, then they won't see any good in making such a sacrifice," Nakoma added.

"I won't let our tribe get slaughtered if they don't stop to listen," I interjected. "Me and my group should go to them and try to stop it ourselves." Of course I had no intention of letting my group come with me. I planned to slip away before any travel plans were finalized.

"Absolutely not," Kiyahe dismissed my idea. "You wouldn't have enough protection."

"We travelled with our small group before, why is this any different?" I countered.

Kiyahe struggled to keep his temper in check. "Because before we were counting on open mindedness and wisdom from the tribes. And no one had immediate plans to kill you. These groups have already made up their mind to fight, and they're way ahead on planning and organizing than we are. It would be a suicide mission."

"You would risk our entire tribe to protect one person?!" I shouted at him.

"I would risk an entire nation for you!" he shouted back.

We sat there in stunned silence at the truth of it.

"And not just because I love you but because I believe in the legend and your death leads to all our deaths," he explained, a little calmer than before.

"Maybe not," I said quietly.

"What?" Kiyahe asked, his eyebrows scrunching on his worry-creased forehead.

"What do you mean dear?" Nakoma asked me, concern tainting her words.

"Maybe it's not as dire as it sounds. Maybe…we're over exaggerating. Maybe the legend… maybe it's not all true." But I could taste the lie in my words.

"Are you saying you don't believe the legend?" Ahote asked me.

"No, she believes it," Kiyahe answered for me, shaking his head. "You're grasping for straws, aren't you?" He directed the question to me, incredulous. "You're looking for anything to convince us that your life isn't as important as it is. Anything to keep us from sacrificing for you." Kiyahe snorted, not amused. "It's not working, Marie. You know and we know the truth of who you are."

"I WILL NOT LET YOU DIE FOR ME!" I screamed at him, my fear overpowering me. There was a long and silent pause after my outburst. Ashkii squirmed uncomfortably, no one had thought to excuse him after he'd shared his news. Now he was privy to all the family drama, which unfortunately affected the outcome of all our lives and which he would surely gossip about with others.

And he would tell others that Kaya was love sick and weak. That she had suggested the legend wasn't true and was blinded by fear.

I cleared my throat before speaking again. "Nakoma was right, love clouds our vision and now I'm in too deep. I love you too much to let you or anyone else sacrifice themselves for me. I have to go, and you have to stay. I can't see clearly if I'm worried about your safety."

"I won't let you go alone, it's ludicrous," Kiyahe growled.

I turned to Ahote then, "Send the messenger boys and ask the other tribes to stand with us. If I made enemies along the way, I made just as many friends and I will ask any of them who are willing, to accompany me to Kalona and the others. I'll travel with as many as will come with me."

Kiyahe must have seen the unwavering determination in my face because he addressed his father instead.

"Father, you can't let her travel without me. The legend says I am her soul-bound protector," he pleaded.

"If you're killed, I'll die," I shot at Kiyahe. "I won't live without you, even if it's possible. I promise you."

Kiyahe jerked as if he'd been shot. I knew it was the ultimate blow. The weapon he'd always feared I would use against him. My love, my death. I'd even tacked the promise on as a means to seal my own grave. Kiyahe's brilliant eyes dulled as if the idea of my death had already drained the life from him. I hated myself for hurting him. A part of me wanted to run to his arms and say yes, let's run away and hide together. But a bigger part of me was afraid for my family, my people, and my heart.

"We will send the messengers immediately but until they've returned, we will not be rash in our decisions regarding Kaya's safety." Ahote looked at me, begging me to take his words of wisdom into account. "We will pray, and sleep, and discuss this more in the morning. A good leader is wise and patient."

"A good leader is also selfless," I told him. And I left then, my decision made, and my opinion spoken.

I had promised myself, after the disaster, after I had lost my parents, that I would say thorough goodbyes to the people I loved whenever I was leaving a place. But now I had to break my own promise and it made my heart ache to do so. I couldn't say goodbye and tell them I loved them without them realizing my plans to leave.

So, I left a young kid to tell the tribe what had transpired.

My future parents to organize our allies.

And my soul mate to pick up the pieces of his heart.

To have courage is to have the mental and moral strength to listen to our heart.

–Native American quote.

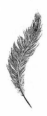

Chapter Nineteen

I hid behind a mask of bravery and surety the rest of the day. Word spread like a tidal wave of what was coming but I assured everyone I came into contact with that everything was fine and that there was no need to panic.

And I convinced myself that my words to them were true. I *was* going to do whatever it took to stop a war from happening. I just didn't mention to anyone that I was going to do it alone.

Kiyahe followed me like a silent shadow as I paraded my mask and gave my assurances. He wouldn't beg me in front of the people, he saw that I was being brave for them and he was trying to do the same. But I knew the minute we were alone that he would try to convince me to go with his father's original plan. And I worried that I was weak enough to give in, so I never gave him the opportunity to launch into the conversation.

Needless to say, all plans for a wedding were put on pause, given the circumstances.

Everyone was gathered in the big lodge for dinner that night. Ahote summarized what was going on and there was a long prayer said before the meal. It was nothing like our usual large gatherings. No celebrations, no after party. Simply a solemn time to meditate and pray for guidance and safety.

I had expected to walk back with our household of women after dinner, but Mahala had volunteered herself and Hiawassee to stay and help clean up after the meal. And Aiyana had slipped away with Jolon immediately after the dinner was over. I searched for the twins as a last resort, but they were also staying later with their father, folding up tables and putting away chairs. I tried to act as if it weren't a big deal, and left with Kiyahe.

We walked in the cold silence for a while and I was grateful for the quiet. But just as I began to relax, Kiyahe started the discussion I'd been trying to avoid all day.

"How can I convince you to go along with my father's plan?" he asked, slowing beside me, trying to make the walk last longer.

"You can't," I sighed. "Your father's plan requires me to leave my home and my family and hope they aren't slaughtered because of me. If we're going to stop this, we have to go to them."

"And 'we' doesn't include me," Kiyahe said, his words a statement and not a question.

I answered anyways, "No, I won't let you come with me. I couldn't live through it if something happened to you."

"Yes, you could, you're just choosing not to," Kiyahe said.

"It's not a choice!" I shouted. We stopped walking then and I forced myself to take a deep breath to keep from starting a shouting match. "How many times do we have to risk losing our lives to prove we can't live without each other?" I asked him.

Kiyahe smiled a sad smile and took my hand. "Just one more time. Let me come with you."

I blinked tears away furiously. "Not a chance."

Kiyahe pulled me to him and kissed me long and deeply. After a while I tried to pull away, afraid of giving into his plans for my safety. But he pulled me closer, refusing to let go.

I'd wounded him earlier with my words. And now I realized that I needed to wound him again. It was for his safety, that's what I tried to tell myself. But it was also for my selfish desire, my selfish *need* to keep him out of danger.

I wasn't going to watch him go head-to-head with any more enemies. I wasn't going to watch him aim a weapon at someone who had one aimed at me. I wasn't going to watch him be pierced by another arrow, or be blown to pieces, or worse.

I wasn't going to stand behind him.

I was going to stand in front of him.

And I had to leave to accomplish those ends. I hated myself for doing it, but I knew it was necessary. I had to make him think I was giving in so that I could slip away.

"Okay," I gasped as I broke the kiss, "Okay you win, I'll stay with you."

Kiyahe smiled from ear to ear and it ripped a jagged gash in my heart. "Thank you," he rasped. And then his hold on me began to relax.

So I pulled him closer and put my mouth greedily to his. I put my hands against his chest and pushed him. He let me push him back and back until his shoulders ran into the log wall of an abandoned house. One that had been badly burned in the disaster and had yet to be replaced.

"Please?" I whispered. My apparent price for giving in. And he did. He was a man and he was in love. And he thought he'd won, he thought he'd have more time with me. He whisked my legs out from under me and carried me into the dark, charred house. He kicked open the door and made it five steps before spilling us out on the ashy, carpeted floor of the living room. There was only the sound of our ragged breathing and seams tearing as we tore the winter clothes off of each other in our haste.

It wasn't like the first time, slow and loving. This time was fiercely passionate, almost angry. We couldn't get close enough fast enough. Even though the pleasure took up most of my thoughts, I couldn't help but feel the stab of guilt buried in the back of my mind. I was seducing him for my own selfish purposes. I would leave him.

I might never see him again.

I loved him harder as that last thought burned through the gash in my heart.

❧

He was sleeping peacefully, that was how I left him. I spared a moment to kiss his lips goodbye and whisper my apology in his ear. But then I had to tear myself away and make my run for it.

The tears ran cold and silent as I raced through the snowy night back to Mahala's. Everyone was sound asleep when I crept in. I packed as quickly and quietly as I could, the tears still flowing. I had a fleeting desire to stop and write letters of goodbye to everyone, since I couldn't tell them in person, but I knew I had no time to stop and do it. In less than five minutes, I was out the door again.

My first thought was to take the new bus Kiyahe had showed me. I knew where it was, what compartment the keys were hidden in. But then it seemed wrong to take it without Kiyahe, and besides, I didn't even know how to drive the massive thing.

So I darted down the road like a shadow, trying the doors on every car I came across. Eventually I found a jeep that had been left unlocked. In fact, it was the same jeep Ashkii had raced home in with his terrible news. The keys had been left in the ignition. I threw my bag over the console to the passenger seat, climbed inside, cranked the engine to life, and put the pedal to the floor. The engine roared in anger and spit gravel behind the tires before jerking hastily down the road.

The ironic thought crossed my mind that I hadn't driven a vehicle since my car had been crushed in the meteor shower.

Back then I had been running away from disaster. And now I was running towards it.

I sped away from my new home, the tears that had temporarily ceased while I'd been looking for a car to steal now sprang up again. I turned on the radio to drown out my now very audible sobs, but nothing would come in except for static. Of course. I cried myself dry as my new home disappeared in the rear-view mirror.

I didn't have the map Ahote had made for our journey to meet the tribes, but I knew the general direction of California, where I hoped my new enemies hadn't left from yet. I had no idea what I would do when I found them. Could I talk them out of war? Could I keep them from hurting each other? From hurting the people I loved?

I raced west, the sun climbing the horizon behind me.

I was many miles away, lost in my thoughts when a white blur darted out into the road in front of me. I slammed on my breaks, feeling the wheels stiffen and smelling the rubber burning. I cursed under my breath, trying to keep the swerving jeep on the road. When I came to a complete stop, I couldn't believe what had jumped out in front of me.

That damn white wolf. The stupid thing was standing in the middle of the road, panting. His long tongue was lolling out the side of his smiling mouth and his bright eyes were glistening in the sunlight. He was my wolf, there was no mistaking it. His fur was a purer white than I'd remembered. His eyes even more beautiful. I got out of the jeep, my hurried escape delayed for a minute. He barked at me in greeting. I walked over to him, he stood waist high to me as I stroked his beautiful head.

"Hello boy," I said. He emitted a soft bark in response. I looked up at the sky and shook my head. Then I looked at the wolf and nodded. "He sent you, didn't He?" I asked the wolf, as if he could answer me. "Fine, you up for another road trip?" I asked him. He yipped in response. "Okay but I'm driving," I smiled at him. "And we're gonna get there a hell of a lot faster than last time. No sight-seeing, got it?"

The wolf barked and loped to my still open driver door. He hopped in lithely, pushed my bag off the passenger seat to the floor with his nose, and sat shotgun with that stupid grin on his face, ready to go.

I shook my head and smiled before climbing back into the jeep and racing down the road. Towards my enemies. Towards my fate.

Acknowledgments

  If you have been following *The Legend of Kaya* series, you may have noticed that there was not an acknowledgments page within the first installment, nor were there any dedications made to any particular people. In all honesty, I never imagined that my novels would become published works. I imagined that they would remain on my computer as old files that no one but myself ever looked at. And I imagined that someday I would delete those files and give up on this dream of being a published author. I am a cynic by nature, and I believed that there was no reason to include acknowledgments or dedications that no one would ever see. I say this not to provoke sympathy or pity, but to explain the absence of pages that are long overdue.

  So here it goes.

  The first person I must thank, above anyone else, is God. If it can be said by others that I have a knack, or dare I say talent, for writing and creating stories, then it can be said by me that I believe that gift was given to me by my Father in Heaven. I have always believed that I am mediocre at most things I try in life. Never the best, never the most talented. I say this not in false modesty or to evoke pity, but to beg you to understand that what I am doing with these stories, with these books, is sharing the best thing I have to offer. My words, my creativity. When I am complimented on my writing, I feel elated. When I am criticized, I feel determined to improve. Nothing else in life have I worked so hard for, for so long. Nothing else has dealt me the most obstacles, and the most triumphs. I believe that God works through me and alongside me as I work to give you the best I can give.

These stories come to me in dreams, never complete but always emotionally powerful and always with a strong message. I take my knack, my talent, and I fill in the blanks and connect the dots. After all, that's what all we Christians try to do. Take what's been given to us by God and share it with others. In doing so, we are His instruments. The Glory is not my own, it is my Lord's. And I will gladly share it with you as others share it with me.

The second person I must thank is my incredible husband, Alex. Without him, you would maybe have gotten one book from me in my lifetime, and not another story more. I started realizing as I entered high school, and then college, that that childish thing we called 'free time,' was disappearing. I believed I would end up as another wife that works to the bone at a career, or at raising a family, or both. That writing novels would become a whimsical idea and that practical reality would swallow me whole. I was faced with the realization that writing even a single novel could take me years, decades, or even a whole lifetime. Or that I would be an old woman before I really had the time to begin such a hobby. But my husband has made it possible for me, in my youth, to devote my time and a bit of our finances to achieve my dreams. And in doing so, I can share stories with you as often as I choose.

While my husband and I share the same dream of being married, living in the country, raising a family, and trying to be good Christians, we also have other, smaller dreams that we try to encourage each other in. Even if those dreams are entirely different. While I don't particularly care how many guns he has or how many times he has a successful hunting trip, I support him anyways. And while he doesn't particularly care about what my characters are doing or what the plot lines are in my stories, he supports me anyways. We want each other to be happy, because that's how love works.

I must also thank my family, both immediate and extended. Like in my marriage, there are a variety of interests and dreams amongst us. And while we may not always share the same passions, I am grateful that they have encouraged me in mine. And it makes my heart happy to see them pursue and achieve theirs.

The same thanks, for the same reasons, goes out to my friends.

Two women that I must also thank are Roxanne and Melanie. While they are no longer my official publishers, Roxanne gave me my start and Melanie has continued to offer help and advice along the way. I thank them both for testing the publishing waters with me and for putting up with my endless questions.

I would also like to thank every English teacher that I ever had while going through elementary, junior high, high school, and college. I was incredibly blessed to have had such incredible teachers who were beautiful women inside and out. I have no complaints about a single one of them. They all recognized my talent and pushed me to improve and excel.

And finally, I must thank my ornery, adorable fur babies. While they make me want to tear my hair out, they also know how to warm my heart. There is never a dull day of writing with them around.